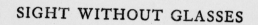

SIGHT WITHOUT GLASSES

SIGHT
Without Glasses

DR. HAROLD M. PEPPARD
104 EAST 40TH ST.
NEW YORK, N. Y.

•

BLUE RIBBON BOOKS, INC.

GARDEN CITY   NEW YORK

1940
BLUE RIBBON BOOKS, INC.

CL

PRINTED IN THE UNITED STATES OF AMERICA

FOREWORD

THIS BOOK is written with the realization that the adherents to the principles of organized medicine and optometry do not agree with this method of treating eyes. That is understandable since their education has taught them principles which are opposed to this theory, and, too, they lack the experience of treating eyes without glasses.

For those of us who have had that experience, this system of treatment is no longer a controversial theory but an established fact. We do not question whether it can be done, it is being done.

The rules for restoration of impaired eyes to normal sight by treatment with this method are simply those laws which normal eyes naturally and automatically follow. The eye exercises are for the purpose of building reactions by consciously training the neuro-muscular control of the eyes to follow the normal pattern.

While we would appreciate the approval and co-operation of the established school, we do not expect it. We are traveling another road, a newer road, a road that we have proved will take us where we want to go — to the state of having clear sight all our life long.

CONTENTS

DISCOVERY

"Half of our funny, heathen lives," wrote Merideth, "we are bent double to gather things we have tossed away."

By the time we are forty and usually long before, most of us have tossed away, along with many other valuable things, the benign gift of relaxation. And with it clear eyesight, for when we have lost relaxation we have lost clear sight.

Watch a cat—how relaxed she is until she is ready to spring, how she pours herself along the floor like cream from a jug when she stretches out to rest. Look at her eyes, brilliant as jewels, keen as a blade! See how strong and bright are the eyes of relaxed, normal children! They miss nothing. Notice how rarely habitually relaxed people wear glasses—even in middle and old age.

Lack of relaxation is the cause of nine-tenths of defective sight.

"I was so mad I couldn't see," is an expression one hears

5

frequently and thinks of as an extravagant remark, but it is, in reality, an accurate statement of fact. The tension of rage has blurred the brain and pulled the eyes out of focus—the two essential organs of sight.

All emotion influences sight, for eyes are like wind-harps, responding to every emotional or mental breeze that blows.

"I stared and stared but I couldn't see a thing." If you stared long and hard enough, that statement would be tragically true—you would be blind. Staring is straining to see, and strain is the cause of imperfect sight. Not the result, as is generally supposed, but the cause.

Nearly ninety per cent of people past forty-five wear glasses either for reading or for all the time. Fifty million people in the United States either wear glasses or, in the opinion of the eye physicians, need to wear them. The increase in the percentage of children who have glasses put on them between the ages of seven and fifteen is appalling.

This book is written for these people, for all people, young or old, who wear glasses and wish that they did not have to. Whether they have put them on recently or have worn them for years and expect to wear them to the end of their days, mislaying them, losing them, breaking them and probably having to change them for stronger ones every two or three years—this book is for them.

It is also for those people who, somewhere in their forties

or fifties, just when they are beginning to know how to live, discover that they no longer can read their newspapers comfortably and that the numbers in the telephone book are beyond them. Watch how they hold print almost an arm's length away from them! It's a warning sign. It needs intelligent attention. The proper place for print is fourteen to sixteen inches from the eyes.

And it is for bespectacled children who must go through the long years ahead disfigured and crippled by glasses, that this book is written. Putting spectacles on children is one of the sins of the world. Instead of helping this small, defenseless person, it *fastens upon him* the very trouble for which his glasses have been fitted.

And, finally, this book is for those people, young or old, who have the humiliation of cross-eyes. Hundreds of cases of cross-eyes have been straightened by following the principles laid down in this book.

It is not for people whose sight is defective because of organic disturbances, such as tumors, degeneration of the retina or of the optic nerve or of the visual centers in the brain—all such cases belong to an eye physician.

It is for all eye disorders for which glasses are fitted, all refractory troubles. And, too, for that fortunate and large group of people who have good or fair eyesight and wish to keep it or, better still, to improve it.

Until a few years ago, there were but two answers to eye ailments—glasses or operation. Or both. When your eyes or your child's eyes got into difficulty, you did exactly what your grandfather did—took those eyes to an oculist and had them fitted with glasses. There was nothing else to do. The eye was practically an undiscovered country then. There were certain troubles the eye was heir to—nearsightedness, farsightedness, astigmatism, cross-eyes, cataract, glaucoma—and somewhere in middle age most people had to put on glasses to read. But what caused any of these things no one knew. Glasses helped eyes to see and sometimes alleviating operations could be performed. But eye men knew nothing that would cure eyes. They didn't try to cure them. They tried to ease and aid them, but they didn't believe that they could be cured.

Then, in the beginning of the twentieth century, a man, Dr. William Horatio Bates, of New York City, one of the outstanding eye specialists of his day, pushed ahead into that unexplored country and discovered something. Through research and experiment, he found out that most eye trouble could be cured, not just helped, that the underlying causes could, most of them, be removed and the eyes recover perfect health and normality like any other part of the body—unless some degenerative condition were present. The eye, however, is rarely the primary seat of a degenerative disease.

Having a scientific type of mind, he had looked for several years with decreasing favor upon the Helmholtz theory which was then, and still is, the theory accepted by most eye men. This theory is founded on the premise that it is a change in the shape of the eye lens that allows the eye to see at varying distances. In other words, one focuses by the changing of the shape of his crystalline lens.

Although a large percentage of eye troubles could not possibly be explained by this Helmholtz theory, it was, nevertheless, the only method of treating eyes for almost a century before Dr. Bates came on the scene with his theory that the eye adapts itself to varying distances not by changing the shape of its crystalline lens but by changing the shape of the eyeball itself. In other words, that the eye accommodates itself to varying distances by means of the extrinsic eye muscles with their varying pull on the eyeball.

If you will look at the eye illustration (No. 12) on page 153, of Appendix, you will see that the eye, placed in the bony depression of the skull with a fatty pad back of the eyeball to cushion it, is operated by six muscles—one on either side, one at top, one at bottom, and two passing partly around the meridian of the eyeball, one at the top, one at the bottom. The first four are called the recti muscles and the last two, the oblique muscles.

When the eye focuses for distant objects, the pull or tension of the four recti muscles is increased and the eyeball is flat-tened out, shorter from front to back, longer from side to side.

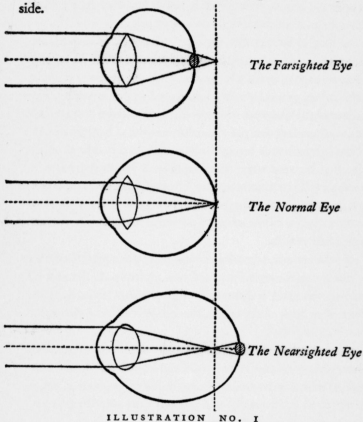

The Farsighted Eye

The Normal Eye

The Nearsighted Eye

ILLUSTRATION NO. 1

The manner in which the rays of light fall on the retina. (Greatly accentuated.)

On the other hand, if you want to read or look at any near point, the oblique muscles obey that desire by increasing their tension, squeezing the eyeball so that it becomes deeper from front to back and shorter from side to side.

As long as the muscles are kept resilient and balanced, the function is performed perfectly and without effort. If, for any reason—such as eye strain caused by bad eye habits or chronic exhaustion, general debility, protracted worry, anything that increases one's nervous tension—the recti muscles tighten into habitual tension, and the condition known as hypermetropia or farsightedness is brought about. If it is the oblique muscles that become tense, then myopia or nearsightedness is produced. If the muscle tension becomes unequal, so that one group pulls more strongly than its opposite, the eyeball is made lopsided by the unequal pressure exerted on it, and astigmatism results.

In other words, when the muscle tension is equal, the focus is exactly on the retina and one sees perfectly. If, because of tension, the focus is drawn out of position and falls either in front of or back of the retina, the image is blurred and sight becomes imperfect.

Proceeding on the theory evolved from these findings, Dr. Bates took those cases that would not fit into the Helmholtz theory, which he constantly found in his large practice, diagnosed them satisfactorily and treated them according to his own theory. The results were impressive.

During the years of experiments which he conducted on animals of many kinds, he proved beyond doubt to himself and the group of open-minded, thinking eye men he had gathered around him that the extrinsic muscles of the eye are the means of accommodation; and that, this being so, glasses are not only not an aid to the eye but a positive evil since they do not remove the cause but instead fasten the trouble upon the eye by (1) allowing it to see abnormally and (2) adjusting it to its deficiency.

While glasses seem to alleviate impaired sight temporarily, the cause of the trouble is not touched. And that responsive organ, the eye, adapts itself to being an invalid with a crutch, although, by the use of a few reconstructive, re-educational exercises affecting the eye muscles, it could win back its normal, right functioning and become perfectly strong and well again.

The results of these experiments were written and published in medical journals a few years before the war. They were presented also to the colleagues of Dr. Bates and to his societies, but, instead of stimulating interest and investigation, his theory was ignored or ridiculed.

Opticians were loth to let go of the old, long-established hypothesis for this radical new premise. And, too, possibly they doubted that people would make the effort to re-educate their eyes. Glasses brought quick relief in most cases, and that was good enough.

Oculists were not interested—taking glasses off of people was, naturally, the last thing they wanted to do.

This lack of recognition of his work did not discourage Dr. Bates but spurred him on to secure additional facts relating to the normal functioning of the eyes. He established a clinic and began putting his principles to the test of actual practice. He was more than rewarded for his efforts. From the start he secured almost incredible results. And they had to be astounding, positive and outstanding, to weather the prejudice and criticism showered upon his work by the followers of the Helmholtz theory.

He proved conclusively that the common errors of refraction—those eye troubles that ordinarily require the fitting of glasses—could be corrected and cured by changing the tension of the extrinsic muscles of the eye. He treated all manner of refractive errors without the use of glasses and, in hundreds of cases, removed glasses that had been worn for years and restored the eyes to normal sight.

Having now proved his theory to his own satisfaction, his next step was to learn what caused malfunction and the resulting impaired sight.

Through continuous research, he reached the conclusion that straining the eyes was not, as was commonly thought, the result of defective sight but was the cause of it—that back of all these errors of refraction was strain. He proved again and again that staring (making an effort to see instead of relaxing and *letting* the eyes see), general debility, nervous temperament, ignorant eye habits and lack of understanding of how the eye sees, pulled the eye muscles out of their normal functioning. This resulted in habitual misuse of the eyes and this, in turn, resulted in impaired sight.

Over and over he proved this beyond doubting. His next step was to find the way back for the eye to its original right use and habits; to discover and outline a schedule of conduct that would return the eye to healthy normal ways and so to perfect sight.

This was done by creating and developing certain exercises which re-educated the eye muscles, brought them back into normal ways of movement and of rest, educated them out of bad habits into good ones.

As his work began to attract attention from the results he obtained, a group of students gathered around him and were taught the principles of normal sight without the use of glasses.

This treatment of eyes without the use of glasses was applied to thousands of people and every type of refractive error was treated with phenomenal success. Today there are people practicing this method in many cities of the United States, Canada, England, South Africa and Germany.

The principles involved, being basic, apply to all eyes and all errors of refraction, at all ages. When a child has trouble with his eyes, the error is slight, usually, and very little treatment is necessary to bring the eyes back to normal sight.

This is no less true for people of middle age or even advanced years if the trouble is taken soon after it appears. It is not age but the length of time that the error has been present causing bad habits to form that is important, far more important than the age of the person in whom it occurs.

In making the foregoing statements, it is well to say again that the treatment is used for all eye troubles for which glasses are fitted and is not intended to apply to loss of sight from degeneration.

In 1920, I began the studies which ultimately led me to Dr. Bates, with whom I worked for many years, in fact, until I started my own practice. There I came to believe that a man who knew how to use his eyes properly would never need glasses but could see clearly his whole life long. Because of the remarkable power of endurance the eye has, one could have young eyes at eighty or as long as he lives.

There I saw hundreds of people from two years old to ninety take off their glasses and attain normal sight. Thousands of people are doing it still, although Dr. Bates himself is gone, most of them under practitioners of this new method, but many of them simply by reading leaflets and books sent out by the physicians of this school.

Yet the world is full of spectacles and semi-blindness and cross-eyes.

In my own practice I have seen cross-eyes straighten, astigmatism, farsightedness and nearsightedness vanish and hundreds of spectacles taken off never to be put on again. I have seen near-blindness cured.

Because I have complete faith in and unbounded and justified enthusiasm for this method of treating eyes, I have written this book in the hope of doing away, as much as I can, with eye ignorance and eye abuse. I believe that, if people knew how to gain and keep clear normal sight without the aid of glasses, they would try to do it. I have written this book as simply and clearly as I could, so that anyone may read it and understand his eyes, may take off his glasses and let himself see.

II

THE CORNERSTONES

One of the most beneficent contributions of this new method is to prove to you almost at once that you are not helpless before the condition of impaired sight. There are things which you can begin immediately to do.

Probably every practitioner of this method has seen in his practice at some time or other what is known as an instantaneous cure—people who so quickly realize their misuse of the eye and so comprehendingly grasp the corrective exercises that they begin at once to see clearly and need only to continue to use the eyes correctly.

A young woman came into my office one day complaining of headache, smarting eyes, and excessive fatigue after using the eyes. I explained to her the three basic principles of normal sight—blinking, shifting, central fixation—which are explained in detail in Chapter Four, page 28.

All she needed was to be shown clearly, once, what not to

do, what to do. Her self-discipline in following the principles outlined did the rest. She wiped out her old habits and was faithful in the new. This immediate cure was possible because she came to me soon after the trouble began. People who have not yet put on glasses or have worn them only a short time or whose degree of error is slight even though they have worn glasses for some time can be relieved quickly and soon restored to normal sight.

Those who have a high degree of error or have had "bad eyes" for many years gain more slowly. Each day they release themselves a little more from old bad habits and take on new normal ones more and more automatically until finally they are free from their trouble.

Frequently people are reluctant to take off their glasses, fearing that their eyes will be harmed and that they may end in blindness.

For many years I have been watching this method work. I have never yet seen harm result from it. I have seen, instead, unfailing change for the better even in cases where the patient was only partially faithful to this method of normal activity and rest. And, as has been said, I have seen hundreds of complete cures in those who took off their glasses as soon as possible and steadily re-educated their eye habits.

There is nothing to fear. The worst that can happen to you is a half-cure due to your own lack of discipline.

You take off your glasses and can see only a blur. Unconsciously you tense yourself with the effort to see. Added to this, perhaps, is subconscious panic over the fact that without your glasses you can see so little. Now, instead, try to release yourself, after taking your glasses off, by consciously relaxing your body, every muscle in it—let it go loose and soft as a piece of thin silk. Now consciously relax your mind—spread it out flat, let your thoughts slide off of it. Relax your face by releasing your tongue and all the muscles around your mouth, letting the corners come up, not down. Close your eyes— free them from the tension all around them, and from the tightness in the eyeball, think of the eyeball as loose and soft, think a smile and let it spread through the closed eyes, think of no light at all in the eyes, everything soft black.

Now open your eyes and look again. Don't try to see, let the view or the word or the object come to rest in your eye, don't go out after it. If you have attained a fair measure of relaxation, your vision already will have cleared to some extent. Always it is the effort to see that prevents your seeing.

The normal eye blinks frequently. It never stares—staring is an acquired habit and is one of the worst causes of strain.

The normal eye is never still, it is constantly shifting, so slight a movement that you do not think of it as movement at all, but, just as nothing that you see is still but has the vibration of form in it, so has your eye vibration. Think of it as free and fluidic. If you have not that loose, free feeling in the eyeball, your eye is not shifting and has formed the vicious habit of fixedness.

The normal eye does not try to see a large area at a time, never a whole line, for instance, just a word; but its movement is so fast that it gives an impression of a large area. When you try to see a whole area at a time, you are straining. Relax, and free the eye, and you will see without strain.

Use your eyes as you do when you write, not straining ahead at all but the eyes on each word as it is written. That is the way to read, that is the way to look at all things, one detail at a time, no hurrying ahead to the next.

As a matter of fact you do not see with the eye but *through* the eye *with* the brain. The pupil of the eye is in reality an empty hole through which light passes; it is the window through which the brain sees. The retina, which is the inmost layer of the eye, takes the vibrations of light that come through the pupil and transfers them through the nerve impulses to the visual centers in the brain. Then you see.

Anything that is before the eye is always in the eye, but you cannot see it unless the brain picks it up.

Lack of relaxation not only tenses the muscles and pulls the eye out of perfect focusing but interferes with the functioning of the brain.

Nothing that strongly influences your mind or emotions

can escape affecting your eyes—far more deeply and subtly than those obvious signs of the close connection of eyes and emotions, such as tears from grief, the bulging or blurring of the eye from anger or shock, the "lamp lighted within the eye" when one is happy.

And why not, since a part of the eye is a direct prolongation of the brain tissue? And the brain, the center of the whole nervous system, is constantly played upon by the emotions.

Nothing that affects your general health can fail to have results upon your eyes. Of all the mistakes made in considering eye conditions, the most common one is to expect the eyes to function normally irrespective of the general health of the body.

Low vitality means weakened eyes. An acute infection such as grippe or any of the fevers, any acute toxic condition, means that your eyes, too, are sick. And yet you will read all day to get your mind off your troubles. Reading is one of the most difficult tasks the eyes have to perform and should not be indulged in when one is ill.

Frequently people, after sickness, find that they have to wear glasses—their eyes are failing them. The eyes fitted in this weakened condition probably never free themselves from glasses—they are so adaptive that they adjust themselves to the glasses and so settle themselves to misuse.

Very sick people never should read at all. And moderately

sick people, should read for only extremely short periods, frequently closing the eyes for a few minutes of rest, frequently blinking, never staring, never making any effort to see.

Over-tired people, nervously exhausted people never should read until they have rested, either sleeping for fifteen minutes or resting half an hour with the eyes closed. Then they should read with the eyes relaxed and for a short period at a time, consciously resting the eyes in between the periods.

One wishes to rest himself by reading. And it is rest for the mind and the emotions, but it takes toll of the eyes. Vision is accomplished by the active, resilient contraction and expansion of muscles and the activity of both the visual and the thinking cells of the brain. Digestion of the subject read demands actual consumption of nervous energy. Neither the body nor the brain is in condition to accomplish this arduous task. The general tone pays. The eyes pay.

Especially does this apply to children. Their eyes are not well developed and are extremely sensitive to strain. Nearly everyone knows that children's eyes must be rested during measles, but in most other conditions this precaution is neglected. As a result hundreds of people have gone through life with defective sight.

One can read in convalescence, but the periods of reading should be short and the eyes rested as soon as they begin to feel strained. By treating the eyes in this simple and intelligent manner, they recover normally along with the rest of the body.

Nervous people, people who, either because of temperament or of conditions, go through life tensed up, using a "sledge hammer on a tack," usually put on glasses fairly early in life. When glasses are fitted to such people, their eyes grow rapidly worse, since glasses do not relieve eye strain and do harm the eyes by accustoming them to bad habits. What these people need is to learn habitual relaxation and then the proper use of the eyes. They could then go to the end of their difficult lives with normal sight and with greater strength and endurance than they would ever have had if they had not been forced to learn how to relax and how to use themselves with less effort and with more skill.

There are four cornerstones to this method of regaining normal sight:

1. Acceptance of the fact that your eye is like any other part of your body, equipped with full power to recuperate under proper guidance. It is not a thing in itself, apart from the rest of you.

2. Realization that strain is the cause of impaired sight, not the result of it. Strain—not malformation, not inheritance—but simple eye strain.

3. Recognition that, since this is so, relaxing the eye and so releasing it from strain is your first step toward regaining normal sight.

4. Determination to learn to use the eye correctly, to win back normal eye habits by means of re-educational, corrective exercises which undo the bad, acquired habits and bring back co-ordination and strength to the eye muscles.

A great many books have been written on the need of relaxation in this world we have made. There are probably as many ways of attaining relaxation as there are types of human beings — amusement, reading, religion, aesthetic dancing, physical exercise, deep breathing, love-making, music, any number of sources. The source is not important—at least no man can judge the right source for anyone else. The significant thing is that it be practiced habitually, that it be not occasional but habitual, that you *get the habit of relaxed state and ways*.

I have obtained excellent results in my eye practice for both general and eye relaxation by one exercise, called The Long Swing, which you will find on page 62, Chapter Nine.

III

STRAIN—THE CAUSE

When the cause of an error is known, one has a starting point toward rectitude.

In the old method, the cause of the trouble in every case was given as a defectively shaped eyeball. In the new method it is strain.

The reason people strain their eyes is that there is only one proper way to use the eye. All other ways cause some form of strain.

There are two kinds of strain, chronic and acute. Strain is acute when the eyes are used, for example, during any severe toxic condition — measles, mumps, diphtheria, tonsillitis, grippe, hard cold, pneumonia, any real sickness. People who "catch up on their reading" while they are in bed with a cold are abusing their eyes as unmercifully as they would their bodies if they went on with their customary activities while running a temperature. In either case they may escape once or twice with only temporary strain, but it is always a hazardous procedure.

Or the eye may suffer acute strain from a blow upon its surface, or from excessive heat, or from exposure to too bright light, or from foreign bodies blown or thrown into the eye, or from caustic drugs put into the eye. Also from excessive fatigue caused by reading all day long or all night long without stopping to rest.

All of these conditions affect the eye's functions, but, if the principles of normal sight are applied at the time of the acute condition, the eyes will recover full normality.

Chronic strain is more insidious and more difficult to account for. The manner in which varying degrees of chronic strain may affect the eyes is infinite. And the causes of chronic strain are manifold. School children often strain their eyes through fear of a teacher who is harsh with them or through worry over a course that is difficult. Strain is caused frequently by improper light, too dim or too strong; by incorrect posture while reading. Both of these are very common errors in the young and much too common in the adult. The ordinary size of type should be held, as has been said, fourteen to sixteen inches from the eye for easy, normal reading. When the book is held closer or held on the lap, as is so often the case, strain is inevitably produced.

The eyes are very closely related to other structures in the head, and any irritation there such as headaches, sinus trouble, decaying teeth, produces strain. Living in an inharmonious atmosphere or environment will cause constant eye strain. Autointoxication due to imperfect elimination, a naturally excitable temperament, chronic fatigue, using and holding the eyes in an unnatural manner (often done by people who have an idea that it improves their personality), any cause of general tension will result in strain and habitual misuse of the eyes.

A combination of two or more causes is frequently found in a diagnosis of eye trouble. The eye is, however, so wonderfully made that it will tolerate a fair degree of strain for years without the vision becoming defective. But, when the trouble reaches a certain point, invariably the eye goes down under its burden, and vision is impaired.

When the use of the eyes is normal, there is no effort in seeing, and the act is entirely automatic. But, as soon as any effort is made to see, strain is produced. Remember that objects anywhere, words on a page, a view, should have the effect of coming into a relaxed eye, not the eye reaching out after them.

Strain may manifest itself as general fatigue, headache, itching of the eyes, inflammation of the eyes or eyelids, and, of course, in blurring or reduction of vision.

IV

THREE GOOD HABITS

There are three things, as I have said, that every healthy eye does. Blink. Center its attention (called Central Fixation). Shift.

BLINKING

Blinking is a quick, light, easy closing and opening of the eye, and it is done intermittently by every normal eye. The rate of blinking varies with people and also varies with the use an eye is put to. You blink more, for instance, when you look at something brilliant than you do when you look at something soft in tone.

Frequently the dividing point between a normal and abnormal pair of eyes is its impulse to blink under a given situation. If the eyes are perfectly normal, they will blink; suppression of the act of blinking shows a tendency to become abnormal.

The action of the eyelids in blinking is most essential to

28

normal eyes and sight. The fluid that keeps the eyes moist is produced by a small gland called the lacrimal gland under the outer portion of the upper lid. When one blinks, this fluid is washed down and over the eyeball and keeps the eye moist.

This moisture has several functions:

1. There is a definite antiseptic and cleansing action of the fluid.

2. The brilliance of the eyes and their ability to reflect light are largely due to the fluid on their surface.

3. The fluid is essential to the cornea, which is the small translucent front part of the eye. Since the cornea has no blood vessels, it needs this fluid to keep it moist or it may have corneal ulcers.

4. When particles of foreign matter get into the eye, the lacrimal fluid tends to float them off, while on an eye that is dry, the particles stick and imbed themselves.

5. In cold weather, frequent blinking tends to keep the eye warm. An eye can be very uncomfortable in the cold.

6. In strong wind or when the weather is very dry, blinking comforts and protects the eye. Under these conditions, one should blink frequently, almost continuously, because the fluid is lost so rapidly.

7. In the short interval of blinking, the muscles of the pupil have a chance momentarily to relax their tension.

8. Blinking also enables the eye to move slightly and thus

allows the recti muscles to make the small amount of movement essential to their well-being, since motion is necessary to the health of any muscle.

9. The circulation of the lymphatic fluid around the eye is aided by blinking, and the eye is strengthened by this good circulation, just as any part of the body is benefited by keeping the circulation of the blood active around it.

Blinking is not an interruption to continuous vision. Continuous vision is the illusion that a normal eye produces, authentic in effect but nevertheless an illusion. When an image falls on the retina, there is another or an after image produced; or, in other words, the image remains on the retina for a short period longer than the image is kept before the eye. It is as if your image, in the mirror, stayed there a moment after you had gone away.

Thus, it is not necessary for the eye to be seeing actively all the time in order to produce the illusion of seeing constantly. In fact, nothing in the body works more than half time or so much as half time. More than half of the time of every organ is consumed in the repair of and replacement of its own tissue and the excretion of its waste products.

The frequency of the visual impressions the eye makes is between thirty and forty images per second in the average person. So you can readily see that blinking does not interfere with vision. It is possible for the eye to blink so frequently that the eye is closed one-half of the time and yet it will see as much as if it were open all the time.

In fact, blinking increases the actual amount of time you may actively see, since failing to blink constitutes strain and may reduce the number of images from thirty or forty to twenty or fewer images per second. There is not a single instance where blinking interferes with sight. It is a fine, natural, constructive performance and improves the eye, if it has not been blinking normally, and at the same time improves its vision.

Do not confuse a wink or a spasm of the eyelid with blinking. A spasm of the eyelid is a forceful, involuntary constriction of the lid and usually involves the muscles around the eye as well as the muscles of the eyelid and is frequently associated with some nervous disease. A blink is a light, easy, smooth, scarcely noticeable movement of the eyelid.

If you have formed a habit of looking too fixedly at things, begin to blink. Blink consciously and often until you have caught again the unconscious blink.

CENTRAL FIXATION

The second habit of normal sight is to have the eye and the mind so co-ordinated that they fix on a small area at one and the same time. In other words, when you look at an object you should localize your attention, fasten it on one small area, not scatter it.

For example, when you look at a page of print, you cannot see the whole page clearly. If you fix your eyes on the upper right hand corner of the page, you can see that clearly, but the remainder of the page, although it is within your field of vision, is much less clear. To see the last word on the page clearly, you will have to shift your eyes so that they are directed straight at that word.

The same is true if you take words quite close to each other. To see the first word of a line clearly you must look directly at it, and to see the last word on that line it is necessary to shift the eye. The same is true if you want to see the second word on the line clearly, you can see it well enough to read it, but you do not see it perfectly clearly when you are looking at the first, and a definite strain is involved if you try to see it that way. This is true down to the very smallest degree of space.

There is a basic, structural reason for this. The only part of the eye that sees perfectly clearly is in the center of the retina and is no larger than the head of an ordinary steel pin. This dot of perfect sight is placed in the eye like a point at the bottom center of a bowl whose sides slope gently—like an arena. This one tiny point has clear, strong vision. Immediately that you depart from that point, there is a tremendous reduction in clarity of sight. There is, instead, blurred, collateral vision. And this is increasingly blurred as you continue out from the center until near the outside edge there is only perception of general shape, color and motion. You no longer have direct vision but blurred, collateral vision.

Since only this point, called the Macula Lutea, has perfectly clear vision, only a very small area can be seen clearly at one time. But the movement of shifting is so swift that the illusion of seeing a large area is given. The images falling on the Macula Lutea are carried swiftly into the visual brain centers, one succeeding another with such rapidity that there are thirty or forty and sometimes more images a second, thus making a whole picture there in the brain.

This ability of the brain to carry successive images and so produce the illusion of clearly seeing the whole object or a considerable area is an impressive and beautiful fact, but it is also the cause of a great deal of trouble. One comes to believe that the eye itself can see a large area clearly, and so misuse slips in because any attempt to do this is to use the eye without focusing.

By "large area" I mean trying to see two words or more at a time. The healthy, normal eye habitually sees only a small area at a time, the mind and the eye co-ordinating perfectly on each word or point of observation with no effort or impulse to see more, just as it does when one is writing.

If the practice of seeing a large area at one time persists over a sufficient length of time, the ability to focus perfectly is lost and the blurred vision natural to the collateral area is the only vision possible; then it is necessary to re-train the eye and mind to look at only a small area in order to again have central fixation without which no vision can be clear and normal.

One can read indefinitely without undue tiring or harming the eyes in any way if the eyes are relaxed and the vision is localized. But, if the seeing power of the collateral field of vision is used, the eye is straining and there is a resulting fatigue and loss of efficiency.

The fact that the eye sees clearly only a very small area at any one time cannot be overstressed. In the awareness of this fact rests the co-ordinating of the mind with the structural limitations of the eye, without which there cannot be normal vision.

If you grasp this fact of focused vision and mentally close your sight to a large area, you will attain this valuable habit of central fixation and find increased efficiency in your eyes.

SHIFTING

The third beneficent habit of normal eyes is to shift. This seems to quarrel with the second habit which is to localize your gaze, but in reality it does not. You must point your gaze, but you must, too, constantly shift your point of vision.

If you do not shift it, you will stare, and staring, as I have said, is one of the worst and commonest forms of straining.

Shifting is a normal function and is normally done unconsciously. The frequency with which your eyes shift varies with the type of demand upon the eyes; for instance, looking at a book or watching a tennis match. The book is stationary and the eyes do not tend to move, while the tennis balls and players are constantly in motion so the eyes must move continually in order to follow them.

But, in any event, shifting should be as frequent as possible. The time required for an image to register on the retina, about 1/150 of a second, allows for a great frequency of shifting with no loss or interruption of vision.

People who are inclined to look at one area too long, and every abnormal eye does this, would benefit both in vision and in eye comfort if frequent shifting of the point regarded is consciously practiced. *Without your glasses, look at a word, then look at a word three words beyond it, then back, and so on. Do this until both words become clear. Be relaxed while you practice.*

Or, if your vision is good, *look at the moon and, blinking frequently, shift your vision from one point to another on the moon. Do this a number of times and the moon will stand out much more clearly and appear in its true form as a solid body instead of a flat disc.*

Shifting is both voluntary and involuntary in character. The voluntary shift is the movement of the eyes by will from one point to another. The involuntary shift is continuous, automatic and very slight. This movement is not visible and is believed to correspond in frequency with the rate of image production in the retina.

When the voluntary shifting is easy and frequent, the involuntary is normal, but if any strain is produced by the voluntary shift, the involuntary shift becomes abnormal also and adds to the eye strain already present.

There is always in every muscle a faint tremor, since muscle tone is not a constant factor but is a rapid succession of contractions producing a relatively steady muscle pull. And, since the eyes are held in position by muscles and all focusing is produced by these muscles, the eyes are naturally subject to all conditions that muscle functions impose on them. Therefore the eye muscles have this small tremor that all muscles produce incidental to their normal functioning.

You can become conscious of this motion by looking at the stars which seem to twinkle, but in reality do not, as their light is constant. The illusion of twinkling comes because the fine tremor of the eye sweeping out to this great distance is of sufficient amplitude to carry the point of vision clear across the star, and the twinkle is, in reality, flashes of vision as the eye crosses back and forth; in other words, the beat of the tremor.

When the eye is relaxed, the voluntary shifting is frequent and the movement is short in scope; the tensest eye can make a large movement, but it requires relaxation and normality for an eye to keep shifting in relaxed condition on a very small area. This is true of all muscles—the finer the movement, the better trained and the more relaxed must be the muscle. When an eye is strained and the vision is abnormal, practice in shifting frequently will invariably give relief from the strain and produce improvement in the vision.

An exercise that accomplishes this is to focus definitely on each word and consciously shift to the next one. A few minutes' practice each day will make this an unconscious habit.

Normal shifting is absolutely essential to normal sight. Loss of vision is frequently in direct proportion to the loss of motion.

V

WHAT'S YOUR TROUBLE?

Nearly twenty per cent of the patients coming to my office for eye examinations do not need eye treatments but advice or treatment for some other condition, a by-product of which is failing or ailing eyes. Most of these people have been fitted with glasses, but naturally without a good result since the eye is not the real cause of the trouble.

More than thirty per cent of my cases have general physical conditions underlying their eye trouble that are actively and noticeably affecting the eyes.

The remaining fifty per cent have eye trouble only and can be relieved completely by confining the treatment to the eye alone.

When you find that your vision is imperfect, before you consider wearing glasses, go to a trustworthy physician and check up on your general health. It is a much better investment to try to bring your general condition up to the level where you walk along as if "stepping to a fair" than it is to invest in glasses and spend the rest of your life with a crutch and many hours of your valuable future down on your knees hunting for the glasses that you have dropped.

The following is a fairly typical case of the twenty per cent of my practice who do not need eye treatments. A few years ago, a young man came to me who had been having his eyes treated by the best eye physicians in the East for a little over ten years. In spite of this, he had been forced to leave college three years before coming to me because of intense sick headaches which he suffered whenever he used his eyes for reading.

On examination, I found a pair of eyes with a high degree of simple strain. There was a moderate degree of congestion in the covering of the eyes, making them look slightly red, but the vision was almost perfect; as a matter of fact, within five per cent of normal.

He told me that his general health was good and, as I had no reason to doubt him, without any further examination I gave him the eye treatment for relief from strain. In three weeks his eyes tested perfectly normal in every way, the feeling of strain had left them when he was not reading, but if he read for any length of time all his symptoms returned.

With the eyes testing normal and no evidence of strain apparent, I now felt that it was necessary to examine the patient for trouble outside of the eyes. On examining his head I found three devitalized teeth and a chronic catarrhal condition. The teeth were removed and the nose and throat treated. These things aided the eyes to some extent, he was able to use them longer without distress but he was still unable to use them with healthy, normal results.

The next step was to improve his general health and his muscle tone. A careful diet regimen was started with special attention given to elimination. This also improved the condition—he felt much better and could do more work. But he was not cured. He still had sick headaches. We had a gastro-intestinal x-ray. This disclosed a dropped transverse, very sluggish colon.

A series of Schellberg irrigations was started to tone up the colon and increase the elimination. Soon he found that he was able to read as long as he liked without discomfort. He went back to college to complete his course and was perfectly well both as to eyes and health so long as the condition of his colon was kept normal. This was five years ago, so it is safe to assume that his improved condition is permanent.

Toxic condition due to inefficient elimination poisons the eyes and seriously affects their functioning. To keep free from poisons, there should be complete evacuation each day.

The importance of the mind and nervous system in eye functioning cannot be overstressed. When one is in great mental turmoil, eye strain always results, not only because of inevitable muscle tension but because the troubled brain is not capable of normal interpretation of the impulses coming to it over the optic nerve. Great fear, worry or grief may so upset the central nervous system and the mind that it is not possible to use the eyes naturally unless one has been taught how the eyes see and what one can do in times of stress to protect them.

One of the commonest examples of the effect of worry is demonstrated by children. Many times a child is able to read a story or use his eyes for hours at home without a headache because he is happy there, he feels secure, his mind is free from worry or fear. But let him use his eyes in a school that makes him anxious or for home work that is demanding from him something that he is afraid he cannot do, and he has a headache. This child needs attention and help with his school work, not a pair of glasses. Teach him to understand his work and enjoy the challenge of it—don't put glasses on him. His trouble is not eyes but fear.

Never put on glasses and bind your eyes to deformity because you are going through some deep, anxious experience and in addition to this your eyes are "going back on you." Of course they are "going back on you"—you are staring probably all night long in your sleep—worried people do—and all your waking hours you are holding those fine, sensitive eye muscles taut, pulling the eyes out of normality.

Merely closing the eyes to sleep is not enough for anxious people. Consciously relax the face and eyes, relaxing the tongue first of all. Repeat the process until you feel that the muscles are free and soft. Turn your head slowly from side to side. See soft, melting black.

Before you go to bed, and in the night if you cannot sleep, take The Long Swing until you are yawning and quite relaxed. Take it as many times a day as you can and as long at a time as you comfortably can.

When you have the general health condition remedied and know that you are under no unusual emotional stress, then it is time to consider the eyes themselves. But remember that a great many people who are well enough to go about their usual activities, who have no pain or abnormal temperature, are nevertheless in a condition far from normal, and their ability to live the good life is distinctly below par.

Somebody tells them that their habitual tiredness probably is caused by eye strain and suggests that they have their eyes examined for glasses. This is pushing a man struggling with quicksand farther down. What he needs is to be asked, "What do you eat? How is your elimination? How much sleep do you get? What are you worrying about? Do you like your work? Is your emotional life all right? How much fun do you have?"

When these questions have been answered honestly, an intelligent start has been made toward the solution of his problems. Not glasses but better conditions are what his eyes need.

It would be impossible to over-estimate the importance of sleep and rest to the eyes.

Now, with your general self diagnosed as to diet and elimination and your mental and emotional state, what's your trouble?

Perhaps it is only simple eye strain, a thing you can free yourself from quite easily. Or perhaps it is more. In the following chapters all the specific ordinary eye ailments are taken up in detail from simple eye strain to glaucoma.

If you are not near a practitioner of this method of treating eyes, you can gain at least some guidance from these chapters. The knowledge therein and the exercises will benefit all eyes, whatever the condition, since this method is a return to the normal using of the eyes.

Keep it in mind that your eyes can get well as perfectly as any other part of your body. You do with them what you do with any other muscle that is unfit—rest it and gently but firmly exercise it back to normality.

The rules for normal sight are simply the natural laws healthy eyes automatically follow. The exercises are based on those rules and restore the eyes to following the trails the natural laws have blazed.

VI

HOW TO READ

Like most activities in the body, there is one way of functioning that is normal, and all other ways are abnormal. This is true of the function of reading.

In the light of our present knowledge of the anatomy and physiology of the eye, many things we formerly thought were harmful to the eyes, we now know to be actually beneficial. Fine print used to be considered bad for the eyes. Today we have larger, better print, blacker ink, whiter paper and finer illumination in which to read, yet the number of people who have discomfort when they read, or who have to limit their reading because of eye fatigue, is increasing by leaps and bounds.

The answer is that we have been "correcting" in the wrong direction, missing the real cause of the trouble. It is not better things to look at that we need but a better way of looking.

44

Most people form bad reading habits, such as:

Reading with the book held too far away or too close.

Reading with the body in a strained, uncomfortable position. For example, the head hanging forward too far or the shoulders and arms tense.

Reading with insufficient light or with too much light.

Reading with shafts of bright light reflecting on objects upon which one is not focusing but which are within vision.

Reading when sick or very tired.

Reading when one should be sleeping.

Reading when one is tense from hurry or fear or worry.

Straining to read blurred or poorly printed material.

Squinting with the eyes half closed in order to see better.

Reading from colored paper that is printed with an inharmoniously contrasting ink.

Reading from highly glazed paper. Such paper causes eye strain if not properly illuminated. Direct light upon it causes glare and eye fatigue.

Reading when it is not possible to have the print reasonably stationary, as on a train or in an automobile.

That you may begin at once to use your eyes in a more normal way, and enjoy and understand what follows more fully, read this book in the following manner:

1. Sit in an upright and relaxed position. The posture of

the body should be so easy that no organ or tissue has undue pressure or tension.

2. The head should be nearly upright also. It may be inclined slightly but must not be allowed to drop forward. When the head is hanging forward all the tissues of the neck and shoulders are under an abnormal pull, the circulation to the head is impaired and strain is produced in the eyes due to interference with the nerve centers that control the eye functions.

3. The book should be held 14 to 16 inches from the eyes and close to the body so that the arms rest against the body; the eyelid should cover most of the eyeball, shutting out unnecessary light and other visual impressions that may distract the attention; the eyelid muscle should be relaxed. With the lids only slightly parted, blinking, which should occur once or twice to each line, is accomplished in a minimum of time, due to the extremely short distance the lid travels. This does not interrupt in any way the flow of impulses over the optic nerve to the brain.

4. The light must be adequate but not too strong. The general illumination of the room should be good with a slightly stronger direct light on the book. The light should be placed at one side and to the back so that the reflection of the light from the pages of the book does

not strike the eyes. Reflected light, exposed light bulbs, or bright objects should not be in the field of vision, for retinal fatigue is produced by every bright light that strikes the retina outside of the spot the eye is focused on.

5. Read so that each word is taken in sequence just as it is when one is writing. Don't reach ahead. If a whole sentence or an entire line is noticed at a glance, as in skimming through a page, strain is produced in the eyes. The proper course to follow is to hold in the mind what has been read and add each word to it. When doing this the eye is kept moving easily and continuously and all staring and strain are avoided.

He who reads an average book in an hour or two is abusing his eyes and is bound to have trouble with them sooner or later. One should either read every word, or, if he is not interested in a paragraph or in a certain part of the chapter, he should omit it entirely. Skimming over a page always will cause trouble because the eye is used when only partly focused. If this practice is continued, the ability to produce a complete focus will be lost and dim or blurred vision will result.

6. All functions, whether of the body or of the mind, are performed through the use of nervous energy. When they are done easily and normally the amount of energy consumed is small. When the nervous system is ex-

hausted through either sickness or the lack of sleep, it is much the better policy to omit reading altogether or to omit it as much as one possibly can. While reading is a relaxation compared to most activities, it is no substitute for sleep and absolute rest.

To recapitulate—to read to the best advantage, follow these suggestions:

1. Sit properly.
2. Hold the head balanced over the body—not hanging forward.
3. Hold the book up toward the eyes, not lazily place it in the lap. Fourteen to sixteen inches is the proper distance for reading.
4. Arrange the light. Have plenty of light without glare or bright spots to tire the eyes.
5. Read easily and deliberately, word by word. Do not scan and skim. In this fashion, you train your eyes to act normally when they read, and so avoid acquiring abnormal activities.
6. Read only when you feel able. When you are sick or tired the eyes, too, are sick and weary and need your consideration.
7. Blink once or twice to a line and avoid staring.

VII

EYES AND LIGHT

A word about eyes and light before we go into specific eye troubles. When there is a proper amount of light, the normal eye may see without strain. In the absence of light, the eye is unable to see anything and should be at perfect rest.

When the light is low, the pupil increases in size to allow more light to enter the eye, like a shutter in a camera; when the light is very bright, it decreases in size to shut out the excess. Thus we see that the eye is able to adapt itself to widely varying degrees of light.

The activity of the iris in changing and maintaining the size of the pupil and the stimulation of the seeing elements in the retina depend upon light for their function, so it naturally is important that the lighting arrangements be favorable.

Sunlight is very beneficial to the eyes. It both relaxes and stimulates. People who live indoors all the time and do not

expose their eyes to sunlight find that their eyes grow gradually weaker. Animals that live in the dark or the semi-dark
are almost blind or, at least, have very poor vision compared
to those who live in the sunshine. It is a well-known fact that
the mules used in the deep mines in Wales become blind,
living underground with only artificial light; while birds,
who wake with the sun and go to sleep when the sun is gone,
have remarkably keen vision.

But it is necessary to know how to use the sunshine to get
the most out of it. Abuse of the sun on the eyes may cause
great damage.

Perhaps your eyes hurt when you first go out into strong
sunlight, in changing, for instance, from the dim light of a
theater to the bright light of the street on a sunny afternoon.
This does not mean weak eyes. You suffer pain or a feeling
of strain because the decreasing of the pupil, the drawing together of the shutter in its attempt to protect the eye against
sudden brilliance, requires considerable time. Frequently
two or three minutes are necessary for the change from
bright light to very little light, or vice versa. The sharp contraction of the iris muscle is painful. But if, on coming into
the bright light, you will direct the eyes downward for the
first two or three minutes, while the size of the pupil is
changing, the eyelids and the eyelashes will protect the eye
from the excessive light until accommodation is complete and

you may step from comparative darkness to bright light without the slightest discomfort.

On the other hand, the enlarging of the iris, the releasing of the muscle, is not painful at all. No matter how suddenly you are plunged into darkness, there is no pain. For example, when you go into a darkened theater you cannot see because the size of the pupil is too small for so dusky a light, and time must be given for the pupil to enlarge sufficiently to permit a larger amount of this semi-darkness to enter the eye. But there is no pain. And, when it is done, you are able to see quite clearly.

The eye can be strengthened in its light tolerance by judicious exposure to light. One of the most effective and simple ways of strengthening the eyes is to expose them to the sun's rays in the following manner:

Close the eyes lightly as the face is turned directly toward the sun. Keeping the eyes closed, slowly turn the head from side to side. Keep this up for four or five minutes. Then, when the eyes are nicely relaxed from the heat of the sun and the motion of the head, they may be opened, but only momentarily, and when the head is turned to the side. The eyes must not look directly at the sun but may look near it. Make no effort to see, and open the eyes only in flashes. As this exercise is continued, and the eyes become accustomed to the increased light, the glance may be directed closer and closer to the sun.

By doing this with regularity on successive days and for a gradually increasing length of time, any eye will be strengthened and its vision improved.

The eye is admirably equipped to protect itself and function under widely varying light conditions. When the natural protective mechanism is used, as just outlined, light will produce pleasure for the eye and not pain.

VIII

HEADACHE AND EYES

**HEADACHE IS FREQUENTLY CONSIDERED
A SYMPTOM OF AILING EYES**

There are over twenty well-known conditions in the body that may cause headache. To diagnose accurately the cause of any given headache frequently taxes the skill of the keenest diagnostican.

In spite of this, school teachers, nurses, oculists, friends feel themselves justified in advising people who have head-aches to wear glasses. The fact that thousands of people who already wear them still carry a box of aspirin in their pockets or pocketbooks for the frequent headaches they have, has not yet made sufficient impression to stop this pernicious habit of fitting glasses for headaches.

Children suffer most from this off-handed, ignorant point of view, since glasses necessarily interfere with the normal development of the child's eyes and push them on toward

53

abnormality. In fact, as I have said before, to put glasses on a young child is to harm his eyes seriously.

When you have a headache, the services of a reputable physician are what you need. Unhappily, many physicians find headache a baffling symptom and are inclined to "try glasses" instead of undertaking the difficult task of locating the real cause of the trouble. But seek one who is thorough and intelligent before you go to an eye physician.

Without a doubt eyes do, at times, cause headaches, but not nearly so often as they are given credit for. As a matter of fact, they are very seldom the primary cause. And, in every case where they are the cause, unfailing relief is realized when the patient is instructed in the principles of normal sight. If the headache is not relieved by this treatment, one can be absolutely certain that it is not the eyes but some other part of the head or body that is causing the headache.

A few months ago a young woman came to me with a history of severe headaches for the past two years. During that time she had had several eye examinations and she wore glasses, but with only slight relief from her headaches. On examining her eyes carefully, I could not see anything there that should cause headaches.

It was a delicate situation, since the patient had been sent to me by another physician who expected me to confine myself to the eyes. Nevertheless, I questioned her on her general health, diet, elimination, amount of sleep, type and extent of activity, because I knew that this woman did not need to wear glasses and that the cause of her headache was not in her eyes. The trouble was uncovered. A simple but complete change of diet cured her headaches and also enabled her to take off her glasses and leave them off.

Unfortunately, in some cases, the glasses relieve the headaches sufficiently to lead the patient to believe that it is the eyes that are the real cause of the trouble. How one can be misled in this direction is illustrated by the following case: A young business man who wore glasses and who had frequent headaches came to me about his eyes. He had had this condition for several years and had exhausted all the ordinary means of acquiring relief. He believed that his glasses were benefiting him, since the headaches were much worse and more frequent when the glasses were left off. But he felt that something more radical must be done about it since his whole career was in jeopardy because of his condition.

On examination of the eyes, a moderate amount of strain and a small degree of farsightedness were found. He took three weeks' treatment according to the principles outlined in this book, and removed his glasses, seeing clearly and normally. But the headaches were still present—they were a little better than when he wore his glasses, previous to treatment, but they were still in existence.

Now that his eye function was normal and I was satisfied that his headaches were not from his eyes, I suggested that he have his teeth and sinuses x-rayed. He had no pain in either, but the x-ray disclosed impacted wisdom teeth. On removal of these, all symptoms cleared up and he was free of both glasses and headaches.

To illustrate further the necessity of a careful diagnosis in headache, the following case may serve to bring out an additional point of some importance: A young man came for an eye examination with these symptoms: headache, eyeache, stomach trouble in the form of excessive gas. He had been examined by two good eye specialists and was at the time under the care of a stomach specialist.

I removed his glasses, which had been worn for two years, and gave him the eye treatment. In a few weeks his vision had returned to normal and his eyes on examination showed no evidence of the former astigmatism. But the pain in the eyes and the headaches, though a bit better, were still present.

Anyone doing this kind of eye work can be positive in his diagnosis as to whether or not the trouble is in the eyes. In spite of the pain there, I knew that the cause was not there. That settled, we were able to explore along a different path. Again it was the diet. That was radically changed and all of his remaining symptoms were cleared up.

These cases drive home the fact that headache is a difficult condition to diagnose. To assume that the eyes cause the trouble is a great error, far too common among the specialists in their respective lines.

The thing that misleads one is that the eyes feel sensitive or weak or hurt when they are used and so they are blamed for the trouble, while all the time it is the cause of the headache that makes the eyes sensitive.

When the oculist puts glasses on one of these cases, he is not doing any more to relieve the cause of the headache than a man does when he takes an aspirin. In each case the symptom, not the cause, is being treated, and the alleviation of the symptom makes it just that much more difficult to locate the cause of the trouble.

If this knowledge were more generally known and recognized it would put a stop to this vicious habit of putting glasses on children and adults because they have headaches.

IX

GENERAL RULES FOR TREATMENT

1. First of all, if it is possible, consult an eye physician who is sympathetic toward this method.

2. If you are treating yourself, glasses should be discarded as quickly and as completely as possible. Weak glasses can be left off "for good" as soon as the exercises are started. Strong glasses must be left off as often as you can, and the glasses must be weakened as fast as the improvement in the eyes makes it possible. Exercising for one month will usually permit a reduction in the strength of the glasses of from twenty-five to fifty per cent.

3. Strain, farsightedness, presbyopia and cataract are different stages of the same thing. Therefore the exercises given for one are good for the others, but they are placed under different headings because as a rule the first stages do not need the more complicated exercises. If, however, the exer-

cise for Simple Strain does not give relief, advance to Far-sightedness or Middle Age Sight.

In each condition, there are one or more exercises that is especially beneficial, but since all the exercises tend to produce normal function in any eye you are free to try any exercise for any condition. For no obvious reason one will receive more benefit from one type of exercise than from another. Try them out and practice oftenest the one that seems to help you most.

4. The oftener the exercises are done, the sooner the eyes will be normal. The more faithfully applied the exercises are—that is, the more they are used on the ordinary eye activities—the more quickly normal sight will be restored.

5. Continue the exercises until the automatic nervous system has established paths which the eye activities follow unconsciously.

6. If the exercises are taken correctly and for a sufficient length of time, the eyes will be cured permanently. If they are only partially cured, the relief may not be permanent since the eye's function has not been changed into automatic normality. In that case, it is necessary to keep doing the exercises in order to hold the improvement. Reaching the point of complete relief frees you from the exercise.

7. When the vision in the eyes is unequal, the eyes should be exercised separately to bring the vision of the weak eye up

to the level of the good eye. To accomplish this, an eye patch should be placed over the strong eye and the exercises performed with the weak eye only. A patch that has a concave surface to place next the eye is best as both eyes are to be left open and both eyes are to blink, and the eyelid of the covered eye must have room to move. The same effect is produced by cupping the hand and placing the palm in front of the eye, making sure that the hand does not touch the eye.

8. Blink, blink, blink. Lightly and continually. *It does not interrupt the vision.*

9. Remember that the only part of the eye that sees clearly is no bigger than a pinhead and is so made that it will see clearly as long as you live if you will not try to see a wide area at once but will relax and fix your attention on a very small area.

10. Make shifting a *mental* habit. Get into your subconsciousness the awareness that your eye must not stare but must be left soft and free to move.

11. Watch how you hold your book, how clear your light is and where it is, how good is the print. Watch until you automatically demand the right conditions.

12. Consciously relax the eyes before going to sleep. Feel the eyes go loose and soft. Otherwise you may stare behind your closed lids all night long. Take The Long Swing before going to bed.

13. Anyone who begins these exercises should read the instructions over again at least once each week—for unless the directions are followed exactly the results will not be satisfactory. If the general principles of this method are clearly carried in the mind by occasional reading of the relevant chapters, the progress will be more rapid and more grounded.

14. The eye exercises themselves are simple, constructive, re-educational, and will benefit anyone who takes them, just as deep breathing or correct posture will benefit all who practice them. They in no way depart from Nature but, instead, free the eye from its artificial wrong ways and bring it back to natural functioning. While they are given to correct the different errors of refraction to which glasses are usually fitted, people with perfectly normal eyes do them and experience an increased feeling of well-being in and about the eyes as well as more keenness of vision.

15. Whenever possible, it is best to have a physician who is familiar with the work oversee the treatment. This is especially so in the advanced and complicated cases. In the simple cases, in children, in most beginning conditions, careful following of the specific exercises as outlined will give excellent results.

16. The Long Swing exercise is essential for every treatment because it accomplishes so much in relaxation by re-

leasing the tension in the neck and shoulders and lower back; and through the long swinging movement enforces shifting of the eye.

It has not only greatly aided and speeded return of normal sight to many people but decreased their general tension and even cured the habit of insomnia. Neither throw yourself about nor move stiffly; flow smoothly from one movement to the other, with the complete lack of either impulse or resistance that one finds in a rag doll.

Many people have to practice this exercise for weeks before they can acquire sufficient smoothness and relaxation to gain the maximum benefit. It should be taken whenever the eyes feel tense and uncomfortable, and should be done five (or more) minutes at a time and is especially beneficial just before going to bed.

If you are not getting results, it is because you are not doing it properly and you should go to someone who is familiar with this work and let him show you.

THE LONG SWING

Stand with the feet about six inches apart. Turn the body to the right, at the same time lifting the heel of the left foot. The head and eyes and arms should be left at ease to follow the motion of the body as they will. Now place the left heel once more on the floor, turn the body to the left, raising the

OSTEOPATHY

Osteopathy, a system of medicine based on the principles that: 1. The normal living body is a self-protective vital mechanism; 2. the power to produce within itself its own remedies and the ability of the blood to carry them where they are needed depend upon the body's structural integrity. In addition, there must be correct living habits, both bodily and mental, and proper sanitation and hygiene. Osteopathy itself is not a specialty, but includes the care of all types of disability and disease —those of women, of children, of the organs of special sense, of the circulatory system, digestive organs, and mental and nervous diseases, etc. Obstetrics and surgery have always been parts of this system.

The most important primary cause of disease is held to be some fault in the relationships of the tissues or organs of the body —bones, muscles, ligaments tendons, fasciae, or other. These faults are not so much the congenital variations from average form, though the influence of these is recognized, at they are the results of bad posture, accident, inflammation or infection. Reflexes from a diseased or damaged part may even pass over the nerves to produce tissue conditions in distant regions which in their turn constitute what the osteopathic physician calls "lesions."

These structural faults or "lesions" result in a slowing up of the circulation of the blood and lymph, leading to edema and acidosis. Nerves are irritated and circulation in other parts is affected.

Thus not only are the vital processes of the bodily organs interfered with, but also the body's natural processes of making remedies to fight infection. This is in addition to the more obvious results of mechanical faults, such as crippled joints and muscles, including or related to the conditions so often called rheumatism, neuritis, neuralgia, arthritis, sciatica, lumbago, etc.

In diagnosis, osteopathic physicians employ the recognized scientific methods of physical, chemical, and microscopic examination, including blood chemistry, roentgenology, basal metabolism tests, etc. The distinct thing about it is the study by observation, by the feel of the tissues and sometimes even by careful measurement of the mechanical faults referred to.

In the treatment of the sick, osteopathic physicians major in the specific manipulative correction of these structural abnormalities. They also give attention to the correction of errors in hygiene and sanitation and in habits of thinking, work and play.

Osteopathy was introduced by Dr. Andrew Taylor Still in 1874. The first college was established at Kirksville, Mo., in 1892. In 1932 there were six recognized colleges and over 8,000 doctors of osteopathy in the United States, Canada, Great Britain, and a few other countries.

Microscopic Type   *Diamond Type*

ILLUSTRATION NO. 2

A perfectly normal eye is able to read the microscopic type held 6 inches from the eyes. The diamond type should be seen clearly at 6 inches and also at 20 inches from the eyes.

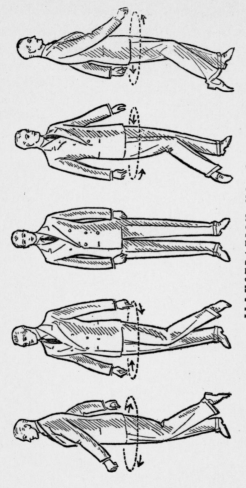

ILLUSTRATION NO. 3

The Long Swing, showing position of head, body, feet and hands.

heel of the right foot. By alternating this action of the feet, the body and head are turned in an arc of 180 degrees. The motion is performed smoothly and easily. Do not pay any attention to the apparent motion of the objects in the room. Sixteen complete turns per minute is the most beneficial speed. (See illustration for position of feet, head, and hands in this exercise.

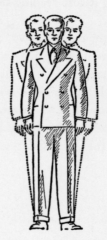

ILLUSTRATION NO. 4
Swaying

17. Reading the Snellen test card also provides constructive exercise for every eye.

SNELLEN TEST CARD

Place a Snellen test card ten to twenty feet from you and without glasses read each letter easily and lightly. BLINK after each letter. Read the four smallest lines you are able to see. Do this for at least five minutes.

Read the card with each eye by itself, covering the other eye without touching it, also reading the last four lines you can read.

Stand as you read the card and sway slowly and smoothly from side to side. (See illustration.) Continue to blink after each letter. Five minutes.

Cover one eye with an eye-patch and repeat the reading and swaying, using one eye at a time. Five minutes. The patch should be curved so as not to touch the eye as both eyes must be left open so they can blink together.

X

SIMPLE EYE STRAIN

When, from misuse of the eye, strain is produced, the eye reacts to it in many ways, just as the body as a whole has many ways of reacting against strain.

It may produce any of the errors of focusing such as astigmatism, nearsightedness or farsightedness. Or, as in the case of simple eye strain, there may be no error of refraction, but there will be pain and distress felt in and around the eyes and at the back of the head, the neck and the shoulders. The eyes, however, continue to produce a clear image so long as you can tolerate the pain.

Some people strain their eyes on only one thing. For instance, a woman will suffer headache or eye pain when she sews and will not suffer when she uses her eyes for any other near use, such as reading. Or one will suffer while playing bridge and not when she sews. Still others are unable to use their eyes at all without suffering.

If the complaint is of one specific use of the eyes it is simply a matter of finding out how one is abusing the eyes when using them for that one thing, and then correct it. When eyes first cause trouble it is usually in some one direction, such as reading or looking at a moving picture or driving an automobile. Later this error is transferred to all similar use of the eyes.

The old method of treating eyes teaches that the eyes are at rest when looking into the distance. This is refuted by the experience of many people when, for example, they are looking at moving pictures. Here the eyes should be at rest since they are used at considerable distance beyond the active focusing point, which is twenty feet; yet a great number of people suffer from headache and eye pain while looking at the screen.

In the light of the new method, this is quite understandable, since the conditions encourage staring because the onlooker and the screen are both stationary. Interest and emotional tension also tend to produce staring.

If one is fortunate enough to have normal vision, the eyes will continue automatically to shift the point of focus and to blink and no discomfort will be felt.

If any discomfort is experienced, it is obvious that the eyes are being used improperly.

Relax the eyes and keep them shifting, moving from one

part of the screen to another. Blink at least ten times a minute and, when convenient, give a short glance away from the screen. This will not distract from the pleasure of watching the picture.

When the eyes are used in this manner, two movies may be seen in one day and will cause less eye fatigue and strain than seeing one movie where the eyes' function is left entirely to unconscious habits.

These cases of apparently normal eyes that have discomfort are a great puzzle to the regular school eye specialist since he finds the eye normal to every test and yet there is the obvious contradiction to normality in that the patient is unable to use his eyes without distress.

The more experienced doctors refuse to fit glasses in these cases, but a large number of specialists feel that they must do something for the patient and so they give "rest" glasses. Unfortunately these bring relief sometimes for a short period but always result in a lowered ability to focus and an ultimate inability to see without glasses.

These conditions of eye strain afford no basis for the fitting of glasses since there is no refractive error whatsoever, yet faith in glasses has risen to such a point that they are advised by some oculists for the slightest eye symptom.

If glasses are given where there is no error of refraction, they produce in the eye the very error for which they were prescribed. This is an inevitable result since the eye is a flexible, adaptive mechanism and will adjust itself to the most extreme condition if given time.

When glasses do not give any comfort, people with simple eye strain go from one eye specialist to another with the most disappointing results. But when the specific cause of the strain is removed, the results are immediate and most gratifying.

The most common sources of eye strain are insufficient blinking and shifting. When these deficiencies are corrected, complete relief is secured.

Sewing frequently causes pain in the eyes. If the eyes will blink and shift, the relief is immediate. It is necessary to fix the eyes only on the entry and exit of the needle—not reaching ahead—and then shifting the eye between stitches, while blinking goes on as usual, lightly and frequently. If this is practiced until it becomes automatic, the relief will be permanent.

Moving objects or riding in a train or car frequently cause distressing eye symptoms. It is because the eyes are staring at one spot too long, fastening, instead of moving freely. Blink frequently and shift constantly, remembering that the normal eye moves freely and sees without effort.

It is unnecessary to go on with examples of eye distress from simple strain since they are infinite in numbers, character and degree. It is sufficient to say that misuse of the eyes is the cause and proper use is the cure.

TREATMENT FOR SIMPLE
EYE STRAIN

1. Blink frequently.

2. Shift frequently. Chapter Four, page 28, explains blinking and shifting.

3. Place a Snellen test card ten to twenty feet in front of you and without glasses read the card ten minutes at a time in the following manner:

Read deliberately one letter at a time. Blink after each letter. Read the lowest line you are able to see, without exerting any more effort than is made to see the larger letters. Be sure to blink after reading each letter.

Read the card with both eyes open, then repeat the process with one eye covered. Do not touch the covered eye; simply interrupt the vision with a concave eye patch or your cupped hand. If one eye is weaker than the other, exercise the weak eye more than the strong one.

4. Read without glasses, holding your book fourteen inches from the eyes. Blink once or twice to each line. Spend five minutes each day blinking twice to a line as you read.

5. Take The Long Swing at least once a day five minutes.

A few weeks' practice, spending fifteen minutes a day, usually is sufficient to permanently relieve a condition of simple eye strain.

CASE HISTORIES

Simple Eye Strain

Artist. Age 36.

History. Patient complained of having a strained feeling in and above the eyes when the eyes were used for any length of time. Vision blurred after using the eyes two hours. Glasses had been tried and seemed to help but did not give him complete relief and he found them a great nuisance. Examination showed the vision normal as to distance but could read diamond type only at twenty inches. One should be able to read diamond type as close as six inches from the eyes. (This is sample of diamond type.)

Diagnosis. Eye strain due to weak convergence of eyes.

Treatment. Treatment for simple eye strain, with The Long Swing (Chapter Nine, page 58) given for general relaxation and release of the eye from tenseness. Also the practice of reading diamond type and microscopic print six inches from the eyes.

Patient reported relief after the first treatment and was discharged as cured after five treatments.

Miss B. Age 26.

History. Severe headache for past seven years when eyes were used for reading or close work. Glasses were prescribed and gave some relief but headaches continued. Two years ago patient heard of "eye exercises." She removed her glasses and practiced these exercises. She was able to leave off the glasses which she had worn for five years but did not obtain relief from her headaches.

Examination disclosed a visual acuity of 20/30—ability to read diamond type at 12 inches. No disease of retina or optic nerve. Muscle balance normal.

Diagnosis. Eye strain.

Treatment. Patient instructed in blinking, central fixation, and shifting. Diet changed to exclude milk, cheese, bread and sugar, and to increase intake of vegetables and fruits. Patient seen one week later. Reported having practiced chart reading and using the eyes in the new way when working. Had been entirely free from headache. No recurrence of symptoms one month after. Patient discharged as cured after two treatments.

EYE STRAIN IN DRIVING A CAR

In order to drive a car without eye strain, it is necessary to know how the eye is constructed and how it must be used. Of course there are people who drive without eye strain, most of the time, habitually relaxed, calm, "easy-going" people, who keep right on blinking and shifting and seeing with central fixation no matter what they're doing, but there are not many of them, and even these people would benefit by a realization of what their eyes are doing when they drive.

Since most of the actions of a driver are controlled by information he receives from his eyes, it is important that he gather this information quickly and easily. Split seconds are important because of the speed at which the modern motor car travels. Lives are lost because eyes and brain fail to gain the information promptly and to act upon it swiftly and accurately, with keen co-ordination.

And yet the eye is ideally suited to the requirements placed upon it by driving. It is necessary for a driver to see everything before him, also the detail essential to guiding the car and, at the same time accurately judge distances. The normal functioning of the mechanism of the eyes makes all this quite simple if one understands how to use the eyes.

Nearly ninety-nine per cent of the retina is reserved for the use of gathering general information, all the information necessary to guide one through traffic. Anything that moves within the scope of one's field of vision is immediately brought to his attention where it may be acted upon instantly and automatically if necessary. This is all accomplished swiftly and efficiently by the collateral vision.

Or one may use central vision by turning the eyes to the moving objects (all objects appear to be moving when one is driving a car—a normal illusion), and then the necessary action be performed. When one wears glasses, his field of vision is reduced, because all glasses reduce the field of vision and consequently the length of time that one has to become aware of any object entering his course. This, of course, reduces the length of time in which he may act. It is impossible for anyone to drive as well with glasses as with normal vision. There is no substitute for normal vision in driving a car.

The field of central vision is used for detail, so essential to driving close to other cars, reading signs, seeing the many small objects, or objects that appear small due to distance.

The ability to judge distances is not a function of the eye proper but a co-ordination of the information gathered in the field of central vision of each eye with the visual centers of the brain. This is possible due to the fact that the eyes, being some distance from each other, see any object at a slightly different angle, and this slight difference of angle, called the angle of convergence, gives the ability to judge how far away any object is. The ability to judge speed is by the rate of change of the angle of convergence.

All the foregoing activities are constantly operating in the normal eye. They should be, and are, automatic and effortless, if one does not strain the eyes; in other words, if one blinks, shifts frequently and uses central fixation in relaxed, normal fashion.

Night driving is likely to cause strain due to the confusion of lights. Glare of lights and reflection cause bright spots and images on the glass of the windshield. When a driver has on spectacles, every bright spot on the windshield is reproduced on his glasses and every bright spot becomes a blind spot, adding to the strain and confusion.

Unless he knows how not to, one strains his eyes driving in the rain or when it is snowing, or in fog or through dust. Also when he is fatigued from lack of sleep or from being long at the wheel. It is at such times that most accidents occur. The difference between safety and an accident may depend upon knowing how to keep the eyes relaxed and normal in functioning.

Very little practice will prove to anyone the practical value of knowing how to see in the complex maze of present-day traffic.

XI

FARSIGHTEDNESS

Farsightedness, or hyperopia, is the condition in which the rays of light are brought to a focus back of the retina instead of on the macula lutea, thus producing a blurred and indistinct image in the visual centers. It is caused by strain pulling the muscles out of balance so that the eyeball becomes shallow.

There is only one way to correct this condition and that is to relieve the eye strain so that the balance of the extrinsic muscles will be re-established and the retina brought back to its normal position. When the focus of the light rays falls again, on the proper point of the retina, the image will be distinct.

Glasses may clear the image but in not relieving the cause, the muscles are weakened still further and the imbalance is uncorrected.

In the early stages of farsightedness, the distance vision seems to be and is normal, although there is strain there. The

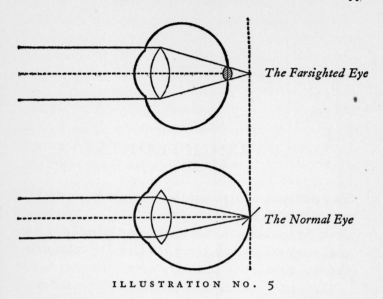

The Farsighted Eye

The Normal Eye

ILLUSTRATION   NO.   5

Normal eye and manner in which rays of light fall on retina in farsightedness. (Greatly accentuated.)

real trouble lies in the difficulty of reading fine print, looking up telephone numbers, and so on.

The usual procedure is to have glasses fitted for this condition and, as has been stated, ignore the underlying cause. If glasses are fitted, they are good only for a matter of months or, at best, a couple of years, when stronger ones are required. This goes on and on, the eyes growing weaker under the wearing of glasses, until nothing can be seen at the near point without them.

The next step will be glasses for distance since continued wearing of reading spectacles will weaken the focusing power of the eyes to such an extent that objects in the distance also will become blurred. Unfortunately, as the vision grows dimmer its rate of deterioration toward the need of stronger glasses grows more rapid—that is, people who wear strong glasses will have to change them oftener for stronger ones than people who wear weak glasses, until finally there comes a time when there are no lenses strong enough to make vision clear. The reason for this is that the brain centers themselves lose their co-ordination under intense strain, and even though the eye refraction is perfect, the brain cannot pick it up quickly enough.

Before this stage is reached, however, one usually experiences headache, smarting eyes, great fatigue, eyeache. This is a most unfortunate condition under the old method of eye treatment since he who has it simply must content himself with less and less use of his eyes and less and less clear vision with his glasses, for he has reached the point where the eye is unable to produce vision irrespective of where the light rays focus.

To prevent this sequence of events, it is necessary to relieve the strain and to stimulate the eye to do its own work instead of letting glasses cause atrophy of the muscles from disuse. All glasses tend to cause a relative atrophy of the muscles.

When the symptoms first appear, they may be relieved immediately and completely, but if the condition is advanced it generally takes weeks and frequently months of doing the regular re-educational exercises to strengthen the eye muscles and to re-establish the normal, automatic functioning so that the strain due to staring is relieved.

It is not unusual to find glasses for farsightedness on children before they arrive at school age, and by the time college age is reached the number of young people who wear glasses is appalling.

In considering treatment, the age, as I have said, is not so important as the strength of the glasses and the length of time they have been worn. The length of time required to secure a perfect result and restore normal vision is also affected by the general health and activity of the individual.

Many people have had their glasses removed after wearing them twenty or thirty years and have been able to restore their vision to normal by applying the rules of normal sight. When the eyes have not been destroyed by inflammation or disease, the vision can be restored, as it is simply a matter of training the eye muscles to function again.

Since it is well known that muscles may be strengthened by exercise it is evident, and has been proved again and again, that the proper exercises for the eye muscles will increase the vision by improving the focusing power.

A short time ago a woman, thirty-three years old, came to me because she wished to stop wearing glasses. She had worn them since the age of three and they now were very strong, the eyes having reached almost the last stage of refractive error. Although without her glasses she had very little vision for distant objects and was unable to read the largest type at the near-point, her chief reasons for wanting to do without them were that they were very disfiguring to her and that she was tired of the bother they gave her. These two things roused in her enough determination to persist in the re-educational exercises.

In three months' time she could see comfortably in the distance and a fifty per cent reduction had been made in her glasses. With a moderate amount of exercise for another two months she had gained for the first time in her life full normal vision both for the near-point and for distance.

The foregoing case is a very advanced one and is cited to show what may be expected in the worst stages. Most cases of farsightedness are found to have glasses of one to three diopters in strength. Hers were of six diopters. These more normal conditions require much less exercising to regain full use of the eyes. From three weeks to two months will normalize over ninety per cent of these cases if one performs the exercises properly and diligently.

Constantly bear in mind the danger and futility of staring. Form the habit of conscious relaxation.

TREATMENT FOR FARSIGHTEDNESS

1. Blink frequently.
2. Shift frequently. See Chapter Four, page 34.
3. Read the Snellen test card according to instructions. (Chapter Nine, page 65.)
4. To improve the vision for the near point, such as reading, hold your book fourteen inches from the eyes. Blink twice to a line and read without glasses, deliberately, don't hurry. Get a ruler and measure fourteen inches to get a clearer impression of how far the book is to be held from the eye. Read as long as from five to ten minutes. Read as you write— one word at a time, without reaching ahead.
5. In order to see clearly for all near work such as reading, sewing, drawing, it is necessary for the eyes to converge to a point. To see clearly continuously at fourteen inches, the normal eye must be able to converge for short periods at seven inches. This function is improved and strengthened by the practice of reading microscopic print held seven inches from the eyes. Measure until you have the distance firmly fixed in

your mind. Blink frequently. (See illustration of microscopic print, Chapter Nine, facing page 62.) Look at the microscopic print for three minutes. Rest one minute by doing Exercise Three. Then look at fine type again for three minutes.

6. Severe cases of farsightedness may require additional aid. The Long Swing is very beneficial. (See Chapter Nine, page 62.)

These exercises should be kept up for a month at least, longer if needed for the eyes to become completely relieved.

Keep in mind that the Blinking and Shifting exercises done before the chart are simply training exercises to help one to use the eyes correctly no matter what they have to do. There is no work to which the eye is put that does not demand these functions. When they are performed continuously, easily and normally the eye is relaxed and the vision normal.

The greater the degree of error, the longer the exercises must be kept up before they become automatic and the more necessary it is that you do them every day.

CASE HISTORIES

Master B. Age 10.

History. Severe and frequent headaches from reading and school work. Glasses had been worn for two years with partial relief.

Examination. Vision 20/20 for both eyes together and each

eye by itself. Muscle balance normal. Retina thin but otherwise normal.

Treatment. As outlined for farsightedness, resulting in complete relief after five treatments. Four years after treatment patient is still symptom free.

Mr. T. B. Age 20.

History. Glasses at the age of six. The glasses were worn continuously and increased in strength, until the strength of the present lenses was plus 6.50 diopters (+6.50). The only complaint of the patient had been that his eyes became very tired when used for studying his school work.

Examination. Vision with his glasses was not normal being only 20/40. Visual acuity without the glasses 20/100. Patient unable to read letters one-quarter inch high, when card was held in the normal reading position. Eyes were not inflamed, and the lens and retina were normal.

Treatment. Treatment for farsightedness. Patient worked two hours a day and in one month was able to read ordinary sized print with ease and his vision for the distance increased to 20/30. Glasses were left off completely from the first day and no trouble or discomfort was felt by the patient.

Fifteen minutes a day is sufficient to give good results in moderate cases. An hour a day is desirable in severe cases.

One month of exercising will cure a simple case, while several months may be required for very advanced conditions.

XII

MIDDLE AGE SIGHT

Middle age sight, presbyopia, is not a disease but a condition, a functional disorder of the eye incidental to age. Eyes that have been normal all their life begin to fail in many people somewhere around the age of forty-five.

This is so prevalent that there is a general belief that unless, around that age, you put on glasses for close work, you will strain your eyes. Nothing could be further from the truth.

Yet this belief sends thousands of people to the oculist, where they are fitted with "rest" glasses whether they need them or not. Even worse than this, it is a frequent practice to regulate the strength of the glasses to the age of the person irrespective of what the eyes need.

And, of course, it is a matter of only a few months before one finds to his sorrow that he can no longer see at the near-point without them. In many cases this is caused solely by the glasses themselves—the eyes become accustomed to them and are unable to accommodate without them.

Between the ages of forty and fifty, there are general physical changes throughout the body. It is a time of slowing up. This lowering of the muscle tone of the whole body is the chief cause of the eyes showing a slight blurring of the near vision at this time. This does not call for any special treatment other than ordinary consideration for a slowing machine.

Around fifty most people begin to dance less, play less tennis, perhaps walk less. But the idea that the body suddenly goes to pieces around forty-five or fifty is absurd. Its ability to accommodate to varying conditions is truly remarkable. Just as it adjusts itself to heat and to cold, to a great variety of food and to a monotonous diet, to hard work and to no work, so it adapts itself harmoniously, if left free, to a slower rhythm of functioning.

This power of the body's mechanism to adapt itself to the existing circumstances is found in every organ. The eye is no exception to this rule.

If you use your eyes normally, they will continue to give satisfactory service for twenty and thirty years after the age of forty without any more difficulty or complaint than is encountered in any other bodily function.

There is, of course, an adverse influence in the nervous

wear and tear caused by the bodily changes around forty-five in both men and women but these changes are not enough to make an invalid of the individual and call for crutches! They ask simply for common sense adjustments. A slower pace. Discipline in eating. More rest. A little less exercise. More conscious and intelligent use of the whole body.

The same is true of the eyes. They do not automatically become crippled at the age of forty and require crutches but need only the substitution of good habits for bad ones. Youth can wander away from rightness and still carry on, but middle age pays the bill. If, at that time, you take on good habits, your eyes will go on functioning in a satisfactory and effortless manner.

The first noticeable symptom is difficulty in reading telephone numbers and the newspaper. This is accompanied by the desire to put the print further away from the eyes where it seems to be clearer.

When the tone of the eye muscles drops, people who for a long time, though they may not have been aware of it, have had barely sufficient accommodation to permit clear vision, find it necessary to hold the print further away, thus lessening the amount of convergence the eyes need. When eyes first show symptoms of middle age sight, this slacking of the ability to converge, is the only trouble in the accommodative mechanism.

As soon as one places type further away, the amount of shifting possible is reduced, and at the same time the tendency to central fixation is lessened. Due to the strain from this change, blinking is also reduced. In this way a vicious circle is formed from which there has been no escape from putting on glasses until the modern method of treating eyes was discovered.

If glasses are fitted for the first symptoms of presbyopia, it is only a matter of five to eight years before one needs glasses also for the distance vision. Wearing spectacles for *any* function of the eye reduces its ability to adjust itself normally to all distances.

On the other hand, if at the time one starts to push his reading away from him, he is given simple exercises to develop convergence, that alone will keep his eyes functioning normally for another ten years.

The greatest loss of the body brought about by age is the speed of its automatic reactions.

This is noticed in every physical activity. The reason that the tennis player and the boxer find their ability on the down grade around forty is that their speed is lessened. Speed is invariably lost with age, but this loss may be markedly retarded by constant practice.

The second greatest loss due to age is the lessening of one's stamina. Any given activity is likely to tire one more, and rest periods have to be more frequent. Heat seems more intense and cold seems colder. These losses are noticed with every organ and activity of the body.

The eyes also are subject to these influences but to no greater extent than any other part of the body. As with the other organs, no special change of the function is necessary, only an understanding of the change. When the eye accommodates, it may not do it instantly as appears to be the case during the twenties, thirties and early forties, but if a barely perceptible pause is allowed without immediately commencing to strain, the eye produces its usual clear, easy image. It has lost a little speed, that's all. Give it more time.

This impatience at the delay of the focusing of the eye is frequently the only cause of eye trouble after fifty. All that is necessary is understanding and the use of the simple rules for normal sight.

This slowing of the reaction time is very marked in advanced age, in the seventies or eighties. There is a slowing in the speech, slowness in the ability to appreciate the spoken word, slowness in body movements, as in walking. Also in the action of the circulation and the function of balance, the inability to get up from a prone position and start off and walk without any unsteadiness in gait.

The loss of stamina is a slow, gradual process requiring no

special attention other than ordinary consideration to the age of the individual.

Unfortunately, due to the general loss of function, the eye's work is increased. One walks less and reads more, attends parties less often and goes to the theater or cinema more frequently. This increase in eye activity, usually ignored, expresses itself in strain.

The readiness of the eyes to respond to the proper treatment is amazing if the case is taken in the early stages.

When one feels the need of glasses or is having difficulty with telephone numbers, simple instruction in holding the book closer to keep a full, easy range of convergence, with a reasonable amount of blinking and shifting is all that is necessary to give complete relief.

For those of you who follow these rules of treating this accepted condition of middle age dimness, an entirely new field opens up. You do not have to accept the failure of vision at forty as have people in the past. You need not look forward to crutches for your eyes any sooner than you do for a wheelchair to supplement your legs. These principles have been tried out time and time again and they never fail to work when intelligently applied.

TREATMENT FOR
MIDDLE AGE SIGHT

1. Blink frequently.

2. Localize and focus the eyes' attention on one spot specifically. See Chapter Four, page 31.

3. Shift frequently. See Chapter Four, page 34.

4. If glasses are worn for distance they should be left off at once.

5. Read the Snellen test card (Chapter Nine, page 65).

6. Do The Long Swing (Chapter Nine, page 62). The Long Swing is most valuable in re-establishing a large amount of muscular activity in the eye muscles. While doing this exercise the eyes are moving continuously and thus shifting is stimulated. It is a good sleep-inducing exercise. Take it just before going to bed so that the eyes will stay more relaxed and free during sleep. Practice it for five-minute periods, then return to Exercise Five. Alternate.

7. Having perfected the swinging motion by practicing it every day for a week, it may now be used while reading the chart. Proceed as follows: Stand with your side to the Snellen chart, having the chart ten or more feet away from you. Now do The Long Swing, and as the eyes are facing the chart at the end of each swing, read one letter. Do not stop to read the letter but keep up the continuous movement,

simply picking up the letter during the short interval the head is turned in that direction. This exercise is an aid to central fixation as well as shifting. Return to Exercise Five.

8. If glasses have been worn for reading they should now be left off. Following the above exercises for a week or two should improve the vision sufficiently to make this possible. Under difficult circumstances, such as reading poor print or when very tired or in artificial light, if the eyes must be used, the glasses may be worn. If progress is expected in improving the near vision the glasses must be left off most of the time, and the accommodation exercised at the near-point without any artificial aid.

9. The functions of blinking, central fixation and shifting are equally important in both near and distance vision.

10. Looking at fine print with relaxed eyes and blinking and shifting frequently is the way to develop focusing for the near-point. Start with fine type, holding it seven inches away from the eye. Measure until you have the distance firmly fixed in your mind. Blink frequently. (See illustration of microscopic print, Chapter Nine, facing page 62.) Look at the microscopic print for three minutes. Rest one minute by standing and reading the Snellen test card, swaying slowly and smoothly from side to side. Continue to blink after each letter. Then look at the fine type again for three minutes. Advanced conditions require the use of diamond type (see

illustration, Chapter Nine, facing page 62) at first, and as this gradually becomes clearer, the use of the microscopic type. Feel no pressure of time, for time must be spent looking at these examples of very small print until the eye is able to focus sufficiently to read them. It is absolutely essential that you relax, that you blink and shift frequently while doing this exercise. Eyes that have worn strong glasses for a long time will not be released quickly, but progress will be seen as the exercises are continued. When one is able to read the microscopic type, the vision is considered normal. Look at the diamond type for one minute, then look at the microscopic type for one minute. Repeat three times, then rest the eyes by swaying or swinging and reading the Snellen test card for three minutes. Alternate reading the fine type and reading the Snellen test card.

11. As a practical training exercise, reading upside down encourages the habitual use of shifting and central fixation. Hold the book upside down fourteen inches from the eyes. Starting to read from the lower right hand corner, reading from right to left, read each word individually and in long words that cannot be read at a glance, read by syllables. Each word must be read by the eye and not guessed at by the contents. In this manner, each word is seen separately and shifting is continuous. This exercise should be kept up for weeks or months until reading upside down is done as easily as

reading in the usual manner. When you can do this so easily that it is comfortable for you to read a short story in this manner, you may assume that the eye is functioning perfectly.

12. All reading and close work should be held fourteen inches from the eyes. Remember to blink frequently and focus directly on each word read.

13. People who have worn strong glasses for years require a gradual reduction in the strength of their reading glasses as they improve their eyes. Wearing the same old glasses will prevent eyes ever returning to normal. Weak glasses may be discarded at once and permanently left off. Exercising for a few weeks will be sufficient in moderate conditions, while several months' practice is necessary in advanced conditions. Practice and patience are all that is needed to recover the vision.

14. Spend one-half to one hour a day doing these exercises.

CASE HISTORY

Presbyopia

Mrs. M. Age 74.

History. For the past five years the patient had been unable to sew, knit, or read without intense eye discomfort. Having tried specialists in Springfield, Massachusetts, her home, and in Boston, without relief, she was persuaded by one of my former patients to come to me. At this time, she was in poor general health and had recently had a major operation.

Examination. Visual acuity 20/40. Retina normal and lens clear.

Glasses. O.S. + 1.00 — .50 axis 180 }for distance.
            O.D. + .75 — .50 axis 180 }

            O.S. + 3.50 — .50 axis 180 }for reading.
            O.D. + 3.00 — .50 axis 180 }

Treatment. Treatment for presbyopia. The distance glasses were discarded immediately. Exercises were performed for ten days with the glasses left off. Then a pair of glasses about 40 per cent weaker than her former reading glasses was given her. These gave her clear, comfortable vision. She left New York for a visit with relatives. The exercises were to be continued and she was to return in three weeks for re-examination.

When she returned she reported that her eyes had been comfortable for two weeks but the trouble had returned slightly in the last week. Re-examination disclosed the fact that the glasses I had given her were now much too strong; her eyes had improved from the exercises to such an extent that she needed an additional reduction of one-third in the strength of her glasses.

This patient returned to her home with glasses less than half their former strength, and instead of being worn all the time, they were put on only for close work. She was able to read, sew or knit with complete comfort. And she will have good, comfortable vision for the rest of her life.

XIII

NEARSIGHTEDNESS

Nearsightedness, or myopia, is a very common condition. It usually starts when one is a child and it has an unhappy tendency to increase in degree as one grows older.

The cause of nearsightedness has been a subject for exhaustive research and discussion for the past hundred years. Many causes have been given as the source of the trouble but each in turn has been discarded for another until it has been generally acknowledged by the old school eye specialists that no one knows any specific reason for the eye becoming myopic. Nor do they offer any treatment that gives the slightest hope of a cure or even a reduction or retardation of the degree of nearsightedness.

Unfortunately, not being able to discover either reason or treatment for nearsightedness has not retarded the number of children acquiring the condition. In fact, the nearsighted cases presenting themselves to opticians for glasses is increasing. When glasses are fitted, the nearsightedness grows worse, regardless of the accuracy used in fitting, and the glasses have to be worn all the time with the strength of the lens increased frequently.

But hundreds of cases have been examined and treated and cured by this modern method based on strain as the cause, so those who have this condition or may acquire it in the future,

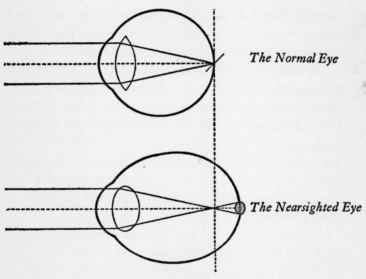

ILLUSTRATION NO. 6

Normal eye and manner in which rays of light fall on retina in nearsightedness. (Greatly accentuated.)

no longer need to feel that nothing can be done about it except to give in to it and wear glasses the rest of their days.

According to the new school of treating eyes, myopia is caused by such strain that the contraction of the oblique muscles is intensely exaggerated, elongating the eyeball so that the light rays come to a focus in front of the retina. This results in the production of a blurred image, especially when looking at distant objects.

When myopia occurs in children—as it frequently does— it is generally not discovered until the child has gone to school and the teacher finds out that he cannot see the writing on the blackboard. Often it has been caused by misuse of his eyes, but some of the most common causes are stomach trouble, with its attending symptoms of biliousness, excessive gas and constipation, measles, whooping cough, difficult teething and nervousness.

The more sensitive and highly keyed children are subject to tremendous strain when they begin school, as mothers who have had to go to school with their children and, in many cases, sit in the room with them the first few days, will attest.

At the same time the child is undergoing this ordeal, he is also required to use his eyes for a longer period and with greater mental concentration than has been necessary up to that time. When all of these factors are taken into consideration, it is really not strange that many children have trouble with their eyes early in their school career.

The conditions are easy to correct if taken at the start or as soon as they are noticed. If taken later, the trouble is greatly increased and so considerable treatment is necessary. And, as I have said, if glasses are put on, the eyes continue to get worse.

A child of six was brought to me six months after the discovery of eye trouble. The mother had not taken the child to the oculist because she feared that glasses would be prescribed. When tested, the child showed a loss of vision of fully fifty per cent, but after talking to her and having her look at the chart without straining, which in this case was obvious, she was able temporarily to see perfectly. If glasses had been fitted to her at the age of five and a half, when they first reported her vision as defective, she would have been forced to wear these disfiguring things all her life and, before the age of twenty, would have been unable to do anything without strong lenses.

Under the present system, this little girl gained perfectly normal vision within a month. She will maintain this permanently as she has learned how to use her eyes.

While an increasing number of children from the ages of five to ten are becoming nearsighted, by far the greater number acquire the condition between the ages of ten and fourteen. This is the time of puberty and the nervous system is under the strain of changing conditions within the body to such an extent that frequently the slightest added effort is too difficult for the mind and body to handle. For this reason, the act of accommodation is not accomplished readily and the child strains to see.

These children should receive the greatest consideration for the tremendous changes that are taking place within them. If this is given and the child is instructed in the proper use of the eyes, the symptoms clear up and the vision becomes normal.

This again is a simple condition to treat, requiring only a little attention for a few weeks.

For the purpose of discussion we divide myopia into three stages. Early myopia up to two diopters of error. Medium degree from two to four diopters, and above four diopters, advanced myopia. A diopter is the unit of measurement in determining degrees of error of refraction.

When glasses are first fitted for myopia, the strength of lens is usually small. This is also true for the first change of lens, but then the vicious progress begins until one ends in advanced myopia. Nearsighted people acquire certain habits of strain as they go along that are characteristic. The eyes move not nearly so much as a normal eye and are held too wide open, giving them a rather bovine expression. This is due to the lack of central fixation and infrequent blinking.

There is no doubt but that it is a lack of all three of the essentials of normal sight that accounts for the steady loss of vision, in these cases, with or without glasses. The only hope myopic people have for improved vision is re-education in the use of the eyes. They may recover normal sight in an amazingly short time, even though the error is considerable, for the simple reason that the eyes, freed from the necessity of focusing to the lenses and urged along in a normal direction by practice of and obedience to the rules of normal sight, once more attain normal functioning.

Recently I treated a young man for nearsightedness who had worn glasses part-time for over a year. On questioning him as to the cause of his eye trouble I found it came on during a period of excessive worry, excessive drinking and lack of sleep. This reduced his vitality to such an extent that his eyes were unable to perform their functions. Myopia resulted. With better habits and sufficient rest, his eyes became normal, with only three weeks' treatment.

Without the co-operation of eliminating the underlying and predisposing causes, it is very difficult to restore the eyes to normal. When the general condition is low and tense, it is useless to expect the eyes to be normal and relaxed.

Medium degrees of myopia, those with an error from two

to four diopters, have in most cases worn glasses for several years. This has entailed the gradual loss of function in the muscles of accommodation, because, as the strength of the glasses is increased, there is also an increase in the strain, due to the progressively bad habits brought on by the stronger lenses. Where this has been the case for from five to fifteen years, staring, eccentric fixation, and not blinking have become automatic and are difficult to correct. Yet anyone with a strong desire can develop, in two or three months, sufficient accommodation to be perfectly comfortable without glasses and for all intents and purposes have normal vision.

The eyes will be clearer, brighter, more comfortable, more active and more filled with expression, the whole condition greatly improved even in these moderately advanced conditions. And the permanent improvement will be in direct proportion to one's ability to replace present bad ocular habits with good ones. Some people are adept at the new habits and change quickly, others have to change much more slowly.

The advanced cases of myopia are the most difficult of all the simple refractive errors either to relieve or to restore vision to. These people practically always are conscious of eye strain and most of them suffer considerable pain when using the eyes. The glasses are uncomfortable since the biconcave lenses are heavy and tiring to the nose, and you see myopic people frequently remove their glasses simply to rest eyes and nose.

Most of these people, even with the strongest lenses, are unable to see clearly. The glasses are disfiguring because the reducing lenses make the eyes look very small and far back in the head. Then, too, in order to aid their vision when they want to see anything, they continuously resort to squinting through their partially closed eyelids. This is an extremely bad habit and one that invariably produces a large amount of strain.

Moreover, the tension of the eye muscles and tissues is so great in the high degrees of myopia that the eyes are usually red and congested, due to the restricted circulation. This retarded circulation is responsible to a large extent for the pain in the eyes, over the eyes, through the head and at the base of the brain. When the strain is relieved—and it is not difficult to relieve enough strain to restore the circulation— these symptoms clear up almost at once. Unfortunately, people suffering from myopia are frequently more interested in relief from pain than they are in improvement of vision— they have become reconciled to poor vision and heavy glasses.

In the earlier stages of myopia, the condition is singularly free from any symptoms other than the blurred vision. Headaches, eye pains, smarting of the eyes are the exception in the first two stages but are quite commonplace in the last.

To restore vision to normal in these advanced cases is a task requiring fortitude and persistence. From six months to a year may be necessary and the exercises must be accurately and regularly performed. For those who are more interested in relieving the symptoms of strain, inflammation, or headache, only a few weeks of exercise is necessary before weaker glasses can be fitted and the symptoms relieved. If the glasses are not reduced in strength, the relief may be only temporary.

The time is rapidly approaching when informed people will not permit the myopia of their children to go untreated. Glasses are not a treatment and no one ever has claimed that they were. They have filled the gap temporarily, giving vision in the absence of any curative measure.

TREATMENT FOR NEARSIGHTEDNESS

1. Blink frequently.
2. Focus the eyes specifically to one point.
3. Shift frequently. Read Chapter Four, page 34, for details.
4. Read the Snellen test card as described in Chapter Nine, p. 65.
5. Practice The Long Swing (Chapter Nine, page 62). This is one of the most valuable exercises for myopia, as the

myopic eye fails to shift easily and The Long Swing develops shifting faster than any other exercise.

6. Central Fixation exercise: Practice seeing one part of a letter best. For example, look at the corner of the first letter on the test card. Now shift your attention to the corner diagonally opposite. Look at the other corners of the letter in a similar manner. Proceed to look at smaller and smaller letters in a like manner. Blink after each point of fixation. In this manner the eye and the mind are educated to a higher appreciation of central fixation. Practice for one minute periods, then repeat Exercise Five for three minutes.

7. The pupil of the eye in myopia is frequently found to be dilated and much too large. The vision is aided if the pupil is made smaller. The use of sunlight is very useful for this purpose. Read the chapter "Eyes and Light," and practice sunning the eyes regularly.

8. The great difficulty in myopia is the lack of central fixation, which in turn causes excessive staring. To overcome these two defects in function, it requires constant attention to detail and to the exercises promoting central fixation and shifting. Tennis is an excellent exercise as its very nature requires the proper use of the eye. For the same reason handball and badminton are good.

9. Reading should be restricted for all nearsighted children,

strictly limited only to that which is absolutely required for school work. The importance of this cannot be over-estimated.

10. Perform The Long Swing for three and one-half minutes (100 swings at the proper speed) last thing before going to bed. This assures a moving relaxed eye for the night, and will yield the most aid for the least amount of effort as it continues for a long time after you are asleep.

11. Spend one-half hour a day swaying as you read the Snellen test card, doing The Long Swing and practicing the Central Fixation exercise. The exercises may be done in one half-hour period or two fifteen-minute periods. If the eyes are very bad or quick results are especially desired, one hour of exercising will be better.

12. After two months of practice as outlined above for increasing the distance vision, the exercises for the near-point should be begun. Reading upside down is the most valuable exercise. This should be kept up for months in the advanced degrees of myopia. Hold the book upside down fourteen inches from the eyes, starting to read from the lower right hand corner, reading from right to left. Read each word individually and in long words that cannot be read at a glance, read by syllables. Each word must be read by the eye and not guessed at by the contents. In this manner, each word is seen separately and shifting is continuous. This

exercise should be kept up for weeks or months until reading upside down is done as easily as reading in the usual manner. When you can do this so easily that it is comfortable for you to read a short story in this manner, you may assume that the eye is functioning perfectly.

CASE HISTORIES

J. B. Age 12.

History. Glasses for nearsightedness had been put on at the age of eight. He had had them increased in strength twice by the time he was twelve, at which age he came to me. He was tall for his age and underweight but otherwise appeared normal. Examination showed the vision to be 20/40—which means that he was able to read the forty-foot line of the Snellen test card at twenty feet. Retina and optic nerve appeared normal.

Treatment. Treatment for nearsightedness. Once a week for six weeks. Vision improved to 20/20. Patient cautioned to discontinue unnecessary reading and discharged as cured. Eight years later I had occasion to examine this boy. Found vision normal, although he had finished grade school, high school, preparatory school, and was at the time in college. Patient reported that for the past eight years he had had no trouble with his eyes.

F. Age 11.

History. Myopia discovered at age of seven. Had worn glasses ever since. Mother nearsighted. Father farsighted. Child a great reader. Glasses had been strengthened twice to bring the vision up to normal as eyes gradually weakened.

Examination. The degree of vision or visual acuity was 20/50. Pupils larger than normal but active. Retina normal. Slight separation of retina from optic nerve at the point where the optic nerve leaves the eye.

Treatment. Treatment for myopia over a period of two and one-half months. Patient discharged with normal vision. She returned for an eye examination seven years later when she wanted to apply for a driver's license. Her vision was found to be normal. Reported that she had not exercised after completing her treatment, as her vision seemed normal and her eyes did not bother her.

XIV

ASTIGMATISM

The word astigmatism is derived from the Greek—a, without, and stigma, a point. And astigmatism is that form of refractive error in which the several meridians of the eyeball fail to come together to a single focal point; in other words, the lines coming into the eye from a horizontal plane do not meet at the same point the lines coming from the vertical plane.

Here is a condition the optician or the old school eye specialist feels, without question, is a deformity in the development of the eyeball. He is supported in his belief by every standard textbook on the subject and, as a result, every patient presenting even one-quarter of a diopter of astigmatic error is solemnly advised that he must wear glasses the rest of his life, that there is nothing else to do.

When I first fitted glasses, I believed this to be true. My education on refraction was orthodox and my reading was from standard texts. Yet, early in my experience, in testing eyes for glasses I found that astigmatism, instead of being a stationary and fixed error, as it would necessarily be if caused by deformity, was the least constant of all the eye conditions. It changed from one minute to the next. It changed not only in degree but in its axis of error. It would reverse itself, for instance, in a very sensitive patient whose eyes tired quickly under examination. I would find it in the vertical plane at one moment and at the next moment in the horizontal plane, or vice versa.

This kind of thing was a severe strain on my belief in the Helmholtz theory. This change and instability strongly supported the theory that astigmatism was functional in character, not structural. In other words, that it must come from a variable source such as the functioning of muscles rather than from a fixed source such as a malformation of the eyeball.

Working from this viewpoint, my experience strengthened my belief. In examining eyes to determine the type of lens to prescribe, I found that the eye would react so abnormally and change its refraction so erratically that all I could do was to advise the patient to go home and rest the eyes and return the next day. Frequently, this procedure resulted in giving much weaker glasses for correction than I would have prescribed from the evidence of the preceding day. Occasionally, after the rest, the eyes showed no error at all.

Most cases of astigmatism are of the simple vertical or horizontal type. This is caused by unequal tension of the upper and lower Recti Muscles as opposed to the muscles on either side, resulting in a relative flattening of the eye in one meridian. This could not take place through any means other than the disfunction of the extrinsic muscles.

When one relaxes and no eye strain is present, the error is lessened or is absent altogether. If the patient is seen when the trouble first presents itself, the condition is temporarily improved or completely corrected by applying relaxation methods and removing the sympathetic strain.

In cases even of long standing where glasses have fixed the error, improvement can be seen on the first application of this theory. If the treatment is continued, the condition is corrected. And if the cause of the strain is discovered and obviated, the improvement becomes permanent.

The muscles of accommodation must be trained patiently to develop new habits and a certain amount of time must be allowed them to assume their new duties comfortably. Eyes resent change, they like to keep their habits. You notice this when you change glasses—you must "get used" to them.

If you have confidence in your doctor, this transitional period under the new method is not distressing. As a matter of fact, the change from wearing glasses to doing without them, ordinarily does not cause any physical discomfort.

Frequently, the patient reports a feeling of relief in the eyes and head long before the vision has returned to normal.

The symptoms accompanying astigmatism vary greatly. With some people, the only symptom is a tired feeling in the eyes. Others have severe headache, gastric distress, or increased nervousness. Rarely the complaint is of impaired vision, which is the usual symptom in myopia. The degree of error has little to do with the amount of distress. A quarter of a diopter of error may accompany the most severe symptom and a two diopter error may cause little trouble.

Usually myopic (nearsighted) astigmatism does not cause so much distress as hyperopic (farsighted) astigmatism. Glasses give symptomatic relief in most cases but, as always, fasten the degree of error so that an increase in the lens is required every year or two. Some have to have new glasses in six months; occasionally there are people with whom no change is necessary for five years.

Astigmatism may appear at any age, but you seldom find it in the very young. It is most likely to occur late in puberty and during the later "'teens." The history of every case should be carefully taken. If full information can be elicited, it is a valuable guide for the treatment. The age of onset is of great importance. If the condition comes on after the eyes have completed their growth (at the age of thirteen years) it is much easier to achieve complete results.

Since the cause of astigmatism is strain—as in all other refractive troubles—it is necessary to inquire into the state of the physical and mental health. More often than not it is found that the symptoms appeared during a period of unusual stress. This strain may be the result of worry, lack of sleep, anemia, lengthy use of the eyes under unfavorable conditions, emotional or mental shock, or physical shock such as one suffers on undergoing an operation.

Worry increases the muscle tension and decreases the muscle co-ordination. Failure of normal muscle co-ordination produces the astigmatism. By treating the nervous centers and releasing the strain on the nervous system, the patient can be carried over the period of stress and the eyes will be found normal when the body has returned to health.

Nervous exhaustion incidental to lack of sleep produces a condition similar to the foregoing. The eyes suffer especially with lack of sleep. All eye symptoms and refractive errors are improved when sufficient rest is secured.

Anemia lowers the muscle tone of the body since toxic products are not eliminated and oxygen is not supplied in sufficient amounts. These conditions cause muscular imbalance in the eye, and the best way to treat this imbalance is to relieve the anemia. When the body fluids are normal, the muscles of the eye can perform their work satisfactorily and clear vision is restored.

Following an operation or sickness when the bodily functions are carried on under added strain, protracted use of the eyes for reading, as I have said before, should not be permitted. The nervous system is not able at this time properly to direct and maintain the exacting task. Muscle strain under such circumstances is to be expected and, once established, it may become permanent. Until the patient recovers completely, the eyes, too, like the rest of the patient, require an unusual amount of rest. Have the reading matter light and legibly printed, the periods of reading very short, and the book held in a normal position with a good light on it. Poor light and poor print always strain the eyes. Using the eyes when a strong light is directed into the pupil strains the eyes. Small print or print arranged in columns is apt to cause eye trouble if one does not know how to use the eyes under these circumstances.

If these few simple directions are followed, the eyes will not be astigmatic after sickness as happens so frequently under the present lack of understanding of proper care of the eyes.

Hurry, fear, exhaustion, discomfort interfere with the easy performance of the muscles of accommodation and the eyes become tired more readily. This, of course, is true of all muscles. If the general body conditions are favorable to muscle action, the eyes are normal. Unfavorable general conditions cause astigmatism as readily as conditions arising from misuse of the eye. In fact, the eye should always be considered as a co-ordinated entity with the rest of the body and not a separate and independent unit.

If you will look on cases of astigmatism in this light and consider the normal physiology of the eye, you readily see why one should not think of giving a crutch to the eye as soon as trouble appears, any more than he would think of a crutch for a sore foot as the first and only form of treatment for the foot. When any crutch is applied to the body and does work normally performed by the muscles, the muscles lose their tone and strength and, if the crutch is used too long, become seriously weakened. A healthy man kept in bed for only a few weeks has a difficult time when he attempts to walk again.

The sensitiveness of the eye is our greatest ally. If the strain is removed and the eye directed into normal functioning, the ease with which the symptoms and refractive error are relieved is truly amazing. Of all the conditions one may treat, no condition will be more responsive to treatment than astigmatism.

TREATMENT FOR ASTIGMATISM

1. For farsighted astigmatism follow the exercises given for farsightedness:

a. Blink frequently.

b. Shift frequently. See Chapter Four, page 34.

c. Place a Snellen test card ten to twenty feet from you and without glasses read each letter easily and lightly. BLINK after each letter. Read the four smallest lines you are able to see. Do this for at least five minutes.

d. Read the card with each eye by itself, covering the other eye without touching it, also reading the last four lines you can read.

e. Stand as you read the card and sway slowly and smoothly from side to side. (See illustration.) Continue to blink after each letter. Five minutes.

f. Repeat the reading and swaying, using one eye at a time. Five minutes.

g. To improve the vision for the near-point, such as reading, hold your book fourteen inches from the eyes. Blink twice to a line and read without glasses, deliberately; don't hurry. Get a ruler and measure fourteen inches to get a clearer impression of how far the book is to be held from the eye. Read as long as from five to ten minutes. Read as you write— one word at a time, without reaching ahead.

h. In order to see clearly for all near work such as reading, sewing, drawing, it is necessary for the eyes to converge to a point. To see clearly continuously at fourteen inches, the normal eye must be able to converge for short periods at seven inches. This function is improved and strengthened by the practice of reading microscopic print held seven inches from the eyes. Measure until you have the distance firmly fixed in your mind. Blink frequently. (See illustration of microscopic print.) Look at the microscopic print for three minutes. Rest one minute by doing Exercise E. Then look at fine type again for three minutes.

i. Severe cases of farsighted astigmatism may require additional aid. The Long Swing is very beneficial. (Chapter Nine, page 62.)

These exercises should be kept up for a month at least, longer if needed for the eyes to become completely relieved.

Keep in mind that the Blinking and Shifting exercises done before the chart are simply training exercises to help one to use the eyes correctly no matter what they have to do. There is no work to which the eye is put that does not demand these functions. When they are performed continuously, easily and normally the eye is relaxed and the vision normal.

The greater the degree of error, the more necessary it is that you do the exercises every day; and the longer the exercises must be kept up before they become automatic.

Fifteen minutes a day is sufficient to give good results in moderate cases. An hour a day is desirable in severe cases.

One month of exercising will cure a simple case, while several months may be required for very advanced conditions.

2. For nearsighted astigmatism, read Chapter Thirteen and follow the exercises for nearsightedness:

a. Blink frequently.

b. Focus the eyes specifically to one point.

c. Shift frequently. Read Chapter Four, page 34, for details of the above.

d. Read the Snellen test card (Chapter Nine, page 65).

e. Practice the Long Swing (Chapter Nine, page 62). This is one of the most valuable exercises for myopic astigmatism as the myopic eye fails to shift easily and The Long Swing develops shifting faster than any other exercise.

f. Central Fixation exercise. Practice seeing one part of a letter best. For example, look at the corner of the first letter on the test card. Now shift your attention to the corner diagonally opposite. Look at the other corners of the letter in a similar manner. Proceed to look at smaller and smaller letters in a like manner. Blink after each point of fixation. In this manner the eye and the mind are educated to a higher appreciation of central fixation. Practice for one-minute periods, then repeat Exercise E for three minutes.

g. Read Chapter Seven, "Eyes and Light," and practice sunning the eyes regularly.

h. The great difficulty, as in myopia, is the lack of central fixation which in turn causes excessive staring. To overcome these two defects in function, it requires constant attention to detail and to the exercises promoting central fixation and shifting. Tennis is an excellent exercise as its very nature requires the proper use of the eye. For the same reason handball and badminton are good.

i. Reading should be restricted for all nearsighted astigmatic children, strictly limited only to that which is absolutely required for school work. The importance of this cannot be over-estimated.

j. Perform The Long Swing for three and one-half minutes (100 swings at the proper speed) last thing before going to bed. This assures a moving relaxed eye for the night, and will yield the most aid for the least amount of effort as it continues for a long time after you are asleep.

k. Spend one-half hour a day swaying as you read the Snellen test card, doing The Long Swing and practicing the Central Fixation exercise. The exercises may be done in one-half hour periods or two fifteen-minute periods. If the eyes are very bad or quick results are especially desired, one hour of exercising will be better.

l. After two months of practice as outlined above for increasing the distance-vision, the exercises for the near-point should be begun. Reading upside down is the most valuable exercise. This should be kept up for months in the advanced degree of myopic astigmatism. Hold the book upside down fourteen inches from the eyes, starting to read from the lower right hand corner, reading from right to left. Read each word individually and in long words that cannot be read at a glance, read by syllables. Each word must be read by the eye and not guessed at by the contents. In this manner, each word is seen separately and shifting is continuous. This exercise should be kept up for weeks or months until reading upside down is done as easily as reading in the usual manner. When you can do this so easily that it is comfortable for you to read a short story in this manner, you may assume that the eye is functioning perfectly.

3. If only one eye is affected, cover the good eye with an eye patch and exercise the affected eye.

4. If the vertical lines are the most difficult to see, practice the Central Fixation exercise (described under Treatment for Nearsightedness, Exercise Six) by shifting only on the vertical lines. In this manner focusing is stimulated in this meridian. If the horizontal or oblique lines are most blurred, practice on them in a like manner.

CASE HISTORIES

B. *Age* 11.

Had worn glasses for two years. Suffered from headache and her eyes became red when going to the movies or studying. Visual acuity 20/30. Left eye 20/40. Right eye

20/40. Glasses for two years and —.75 cylinders in front of each eye.

Treatments given for three weeks, one each week. Patient discharged with normal sight. There has been no recurrence of any form of eye trouble for the past seven years.

Age 14.

This child could not see the board when she was sent to school. Several specialists tested her eyes and prescribed glasses. Glasses were changed frequently as the eyes grew weaker. Child was strong and healthy, and slightly overweight.

Examination. Glasses very strong (O. D. + 2.50 Cyl.); (O. S. + 4.00 Cyl.).

Vision with glasses only 20/40.

Vision without glasses 20/100.

Child squinted her eyes and stared when trying to read the chart.

Treatment given as outlined for astigmatism. Glasses were left off and the exercises done regularly for three months. When discharged, vision was nearly normal (20/30), without glasses. The eyes appeared normal and the child used them in a normal manner, giving her a greatly improved appearance and personality. Her vision will continue to improve without direction if her exercises are kept up.

XV

CROSS-EYES

Strabismus or cross-eyes, is one of the most distressing of eye troubles. The child who is unfortunate enough to have this error starts life with a tremendous handicap, and, as he grows older, his entire personality is warped and perverted by this most unhappy of eye plights.

Cross-eyes is caused by the failure of the muscles of the eyes to hold the eyeball in such a way that each eye is directed toward the same point at the same time. When this happens in a baby a few weeks or a few months old, it should cause no great concern, since in all probability it means nothing more than that the muscles have not developed co-ordination any more than the hand or arm muscles have. But care should be taken not to allow the baby to strain his eyes. He must be kept from lights that are too bright, and the crib should be placed in the room in such a position that the child can see people approaching him without having to look to one side continually. He should not have things thrust close to his eyes to attract his attention. Nor should there be any sudden movements around him; accommodation is very weak and poorly developed in a baby, and sudden movement demands too violent accommodation.

Two images are carried into the brain, one from each eye, but in the mind there will be only one image. To produce this is a complex and complicated function of the nervous system. As the nervous reactions of a baby are very simple when he is born, it is some time before the more complex reactions develop. A baby cannot be said to see in any sense that an adult sees. Seeing in an adult involves thinking, comparing the thing in the mind with previous visual pictures— this is automatic and unconscious, but it is, none the less, an integral part of seeing.

A baby must experience a great number and variety of visual impressions before this faculty becomes really active. When it is that the child actually begins to see in an adult sense is not known; some scientists place the age as early as six months while others place it as late as four years. The more recent investigators lead us to believe that the child has this function of making a single mental picture from the two eyes before the age of one and one-half years and, sometimes, before the age of one year.

This ability of the mind to take two images and make them

into one is called the fusion faculty. Before this faculty is developed, the child sees with either eye indiscriminately. For this reason he should be so handled that each eye will have a fair amount of exercise or he will become accustomed to using only one eye. If this happens, the other eye loses its urge to see and no longer directs itself toward the object at which the seeing eye is looking.

When he reaches the age of one or one and a half years, when the fusion faculty becomes active, if he has a habit of seeing with only one eye, he develops an ability to suppress the image from the crossing eye. Because of this, a cross-eyed person has, for all practical purposes, only one-eyed vision, the other eye is entirely dormant and does not see at all.

The foregoing is the usual type of cross-eyes. Another type is where the child has good vision in each eye and uses both eyes but, due to the lack of fusion, is not able to use both eyes at the same time. This is known as a case of alternating squint or cross-eyes.

Alternating squint is found in children who are highly strung, or are in delicate health or are, for some reason, excessively nervous. If these children are cured of their ill-health, the fusion faculty will in all probability develop normally.

The old school oculists are not agreed as to the best procedure to follow in cross-eye cases. Some doctors prescribe glasses at a very early age and you see children two years old wearing strong glasses. Other doctors prescribe drops to put in the good eye to blur the vision and so force the weaker eye into action. Still others do not take any action at all—they wait to see if the child will grow out of this condition and if he doesn't, then they operate.

It is obvious to any observer that none of these methods has produced the desired results as there are a distressing number of cross-eyed people in the world, and there seem to be an increasing number of children so afflicted.

Cross-eyes may occur at any age; from infantile paralysis affecting the eye muscles; from sudden fright; blows on the head causing loss of function of one or more eye muscles; rare, degenerative diseases of the brain.

One of my first cases of cross-eyes was a little girl about seven years old who had been cross-eyed for six months. The condition was brought about by a severe strain placed not only upon her whole nervous system but definitely upon her eyes when a dog jumped up on her and she thought that he was going to bite her eyes. The fright caused her eyes to cross and they stayed that way. I expected this to be a very easy case to clear up, but it did not prove to be so. It took over two months of regular, re-educational exercises to restore normal function and straighten that child's eyes.

A similar case is of a woman of thirty-eight who had been

in an automobile accident. The car she was in was struck on the right side. Although she was not in any way hurt or jarred, since the accident was a minor one, her right eye turned out and remained that way. The cause was fear and nervous shock—she had been afraid that glass would cut her eye. Four months after the accident, and after seeing three specialists without results, she came to see me. Five treatments by the modern method completely cured her.

Some cases of accident require no local treatment to the eyes. If one is suffering from concussion of the brain or fracture of the skull, the eye symptoms usually clear up with the rest that is always prescribed for the head injury.

Operations for cross-eyes are very uncertain. Some surgeons operate on children as early as six years of age, while others wait until they are twelve or fourteen before operating. In any event less than half the cases are successful one year after the operation and in almost every case the child must wear heavy glasses afterward.

The principles of relaxation and relief from strain have been singularly successful in curing cross-eyed children. Many of them have been released both from the necessity of wearing glasses and from the crossed eyes by only a few weeks' treatment.

Children who have weak fusion or very poor vision in one eye usually require treatment for a much longer time in order to develop normal sight. I have never had a case of cross-eyes that has not been improved.

Some children, whose one eye turns in badly, are benefited at once by relieving the strain; others, although helped, benefit most when a reasonable amount of exercise is followed by an operation to balance the muscles of the eye. They are then given a short series of exercises, after the operation, to restore the eyes to complete normal vision. This is, then, a very good procedure in severe cases and cases of long standing, because the muscles are so out of balance that the amount of exercise necessary to develop normality is too much to ask of a child.

When the exercises have been used in conjunction with operation, the very worst cases have had a most happy result.

If the case is one of alternating squint, an effort to secure fusion is made through the use of the eye patch described under "General Rules For Treatment." When the eyes are perfectly relaxed, they appear absolutely straight. But when these children with an alternating squint are tired, the eyes cross. I have several of these children whose eyes, after treatment, see perfectly and, in fact, appear perfect most of the time, but due to weak fusion, the eyes will not stay in position when the child is over-tired or sick. Operative procedure or fitting glasses does not offer much in these cases as the eyes are already as straight as any surgeon can hope to make them, and their failure to stay straight all the time is the under-developed fusion center in the brain. These children need an unusual amount of rest and freedom from excitement.

It is only in the past six or seven years that any real effort has been made to develop fusion as very little is known about its production in the nervous connections of the brain centers. Clinics are now being established to study this most essential function.

Many of the cases that have not found relief in glasses or operation present no serious problem to the present system of treating cross-eyes. Every child should be given a chance for normal sight by having the modern methods of relaxation tried as soon as possible. Those with long-standing conditions should receive every encouragement to look into this different system. They may be astonished to find that their trouble presents to it no difficulty.

In the past five months, I have treated four cases of cross-eyes in adults. All were over twenty years of age. All wore strong glasses. One had been operated upon twice unsuccessfully. In every case the glasses were removed, the eyes straightened and the vision brought up to normal.

TREATMENT FOR CROSS-EYES

1. In very young children the only treatment necessary for cross-eyes is a comfortable eye patch over the fixing eye (the eye that is not crossed), in order to force the child to use the crossing eye.

By forcing him to use the crossing eye, you overcome its loss of sight, since disuse of an eye always causes loss of function and dim vision. Thus both eyes become accustomed to seeing and normal development of vision is greatly aided. In many cases where this procedure is followed as soon as the trouble is noticed, the eyes co-ordinate and the condition requires no further attention.

If the child is very young and the patch upsets him and makes him cry, remove it at the end of five minutes. As he becomes accustomed to it, the patch should be left on for increasing lengths of time until it can be left in place all day. It is well to associate the wearing of the patch with some pleasure, toys that he is especially fond of, and that he uses only when the patch is on, or certain songs he likes, anything that pleases him and that happens to him only when he wears the patch. Some children will keep the patch on contentedly if the mother or nurse will wear one to keep them company.

2. In children where the wearing of the patch has not been sufficient to correct the condition, or where glasses have been

worn and the condition still persists, the exercises outlined under farsightedness should be given the crossing eye while a patch is worn over the fixing eye. The exercises for farsightedness should be used for farsighted eyes and the directions for nearsightedness should be followed if the crossing eye is nearsighted. In either case, the exercises should be gone through regularly with the patch on and with the patch off.

3. When doing the Long Swing, always stand with the crossing eye next the card, so that its tendency is to look to the opposite side from its crossed position. The eye must be used with blinking, central fixation and shifting. The importance of these rules cannot be over-estimated.

4. Lack of fusion is the great difficulty with cross-eyes. The ability of the nervous system to make the two images into one is called fusion. And the success of any treatment depends upon the regaining of this function. To use both eyes and to see clearly a single image when there are really two images, one in each eye, is a complex function of the nervous system (see illustration of the eye nerve tracts). If the eyes are relaxed and used without strain, the conditions are favorable to the development of fusion. When the person is not well or unduly nervous or tired or uses the eyes improperly so that strain is produced, the fusion faculty is carried on poorly or not at all.

3. The exercises advised in the preceding paragraph are

for improvement in the general use of the eyes and for the development of increased visual strength in the weak eye. Having improved the manner in which the eyes are used and increased the vision in the weak eye, specific exercises may now be given for training the fusion faculty. Without an active fusion center, no pair of eyes can be kept perfectly straight. The urge to see the same spot at the same time by the two eyes is what directs the eyes and co-ordinates them. The angle of convergence of the eyes makes it possible to judge distances that would be impossible with one-eyed vision.

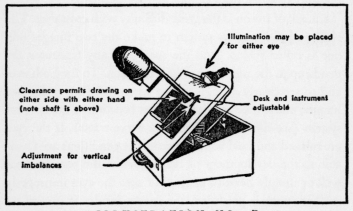

ILLUSTRATION NO. 7

Eyescope for correcting upward or downward deviation of one eye.

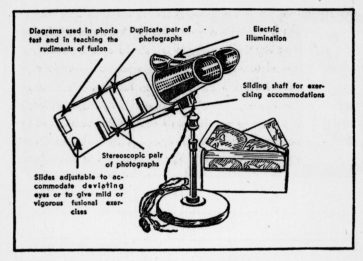

Diagrams used in phoria test and in teaching the rudiments of fusion

Duplicate pair of photographs

Electric illumination

Sliding shaft for exercising accommodations

Stereoscopic pair of photographs

Slides adjustable to accommodate deviating eyes or to give mild or vigorous fusional exercises

ILLUSTRATION NO. 8
Eyescope for correcting lateral deviation of one eye.

To stimulate the fusion and develop the faculty to a normal degree, special equipment is necessary. The eyescope is an adaptation of the old-fashioned stereoscope in which special cards are used. The cards are made with and without perspective and, in this manner, a clear contrast is made in the mind of the patient.

The two eyes are stimulated to see together by placing a part of a familiar object before one eye and the remainder of

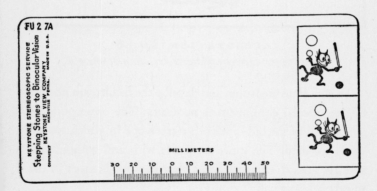

ILLUSTRATION NO. 9
Cards used in Eyescope (see Illustration 8, page 132)

the object before the other eye. To see the whole object it must be seen with both eyes at once through the function of the fusion center. The instrument is adjustable to any type of cross-eyed condition so that the objects to be seen can be placed in the most suitable position for that pair of eyes. Once fusion is established, practice with the eyescope will develop it to a normal degree. The instrument and the special cards that accompany it are a most valuable aid for training crossed eyes. This instrument represents the greatest non-surgical advance in the past fifty years for treating this condition.

The accompanying illustrations will give some idea of the manner in which it is used and the tremendous possibilities it has for benefiting crossed eyes.

These eyes always require advice and must be placed under the care of someone familiar with this method.

CASE HISTORY

A. Age 14.

History. Child had been cross-eyed from birth. The eyes were badly crossed if the child was sick or very tired and not so badly crossed when she was rested and well. The crossing had been much worse at the age of five when she started school. Glasses had been fitted at the age of two, and they seemed to keep the eyes straighter. Glasses were increased in strength from time to time. Child had a mastoid operation which did not heal normally and the eyes became worse.

Examination disclosed a fairly well nourished child, tall for her age, and the left eye turned in toward her nose. Vision in straight eye good with glasses on but poor without glasses. Crossed eye vision poor with glasses and very poor without.

Glasses. + 3.50 — 1.50 C. 90.
            + 3.50 — 1.50 C. 90.

The left mastoid incision had failed to heal and was covered with dressing.

Treatment as outlined for cross-eyes. Glasses were left off and eye training commenced. Vision improved and eyes were noticeably straighter. After three months of work the eyes were straightened, the vision was normal. The health of the child was improved and she was operated on to close the mastoid incision. Operation was successful and mastoid healed normally. At the present time, eight years later, the eyes are normal, vision normal and comfortable.

XVI

CATARACT

Following the retrogressive stages of a misused eye, it is interesting to note that even so severe a condition as cataract has its beginning in strain. Cataract is nothing but the result of long, continuous, severe strain.

When an eye that is normal begins to strain and goes beyond the point of simple eye strain, it unfailingly brings about some error of refraction. If the straining is produced when reading or using the eye at a near point, farsightedness is caused. If this is continued, presbyopia or the dim vision of middle age is produced. If this strain is continued or increased, cataract is brought about. Wearing glasses for the initial stage of simple strain will increase the strain and hasten the advent of presbyopia. And wearing stronger glasses for presbyopia will increase the possibility of cataract.

There is always a severe strain produced when strong

glasses are worn continuously or bifocal glasses are worn for any length of time.

Contrary to popular beliefs, cataract is not a growth. It is a condition of the crystalline lens which becomes opaque and does not allow the light rays to pass through to the retina. Any part of the lens may be affected. Sometimes the opacity is in the center, causing loss of vision very early in the condition; at other times the opacity is at the periphery and the vision is not materially affected until very late in its retrogression.

And then there are cases where the opacities appear as small flaky spots in any part of the lens and cause spotty irregularities in the visual field.

To understand where a cataract really is and what causes it, you must know the structure of the eye. If you will look at the sketch of the eye on page 157 you will realize that a cataract cannot be seen except by an eye specialist, because the crystalline lens is so far back in the eye.

The crystalline lens is a transparent, colorless biconvex disc measuring five millimeters in thickness and nine millimeters in diameter. It is suspended by its ligament and divides the aqueous from the vitreous humor. The iris lies immediately in front of the lens.

It is made up of concentric layers, very like the layers in an onion. Between these layers are small lymph channels for fluid to pass into the substance of the lens.

When the strain in the eye is sufficient to cause compression of the lens, the lymph fluid is not able to pass through but is pressed out and the lens becomes hard and dry. If this dryness goes to the point of the layers separating, this irregularity makes the lens opaque.

The necessity of a perfectly uniform structure in the lens may be illustrated in two ways. If you take a pail of clear water and look into it when it is at rest, anything in the bottom can be seen clearly. But if there is a slight ripple made on the top of the water, although the water is as clear as ever, you are unable to see the bottom. The irregularity in the water makes it opaque.

In the same way bathroom windows may be made so no clear images pass through them. The glass may be perfectly clear, but if one side is irregular in its surface, the light rays are broken up and no clear image is transmitted.

This is exactly what happens when irregularity occurs in the lens.

While most cataracts come in the middle aged and the old, cataracts may be formed immediately at any age from a blow in the eye and are quite common in boxers. Even children can have them from blows upon the eye. The fact that compression may cause cataract can be demonstrated with fresh animal eyes. If the fresh animal eye is compressed around the periphery, the lens becomes opaque. When the pressure is relieved, the lens becomes clear again.

As in the case of any eye strain, the treatment for cataract is to normalize the eye functions. If the strain of the eye can be reduced, the tension is also reduced. This reduction in tension reduces the pressure on the crystalline lens and the fluid is allowed to pass through the lymph channels and keep the lens properly lubricated so that the layers do not separate. Thus the cause of the separation of the layers of the lens is done away with and the progress of the cataract is arrested.

Once the layers of the lens have been separated, they do not tend to re-establish themselves completely, and it is necessary to train the person to see without strain, even though the field of vision is not entirely clear. This is no more difficult than training a person to see through spectacles that are not clear or through a window that is misty.

Many of the cases of cataract still show evidence of the injury of the lens, yet can pass any examination for normal vision since they see normally at both the near and the distant points.

I treated a case where the lens was uniformly opaque and in a condition ripe for operation, yet the treatment permitted the patient to see sufficiently well to go about and to attend to familiar duties. Ordinarily when cataracts have progressed to the operable stage, it is best to go through with the operation, which in many cases gives a good degree of vision. In the case cited above, the patient had had one eye operated upon but the operation had been a failure and the eye was blind. Whenever the operation is a failure, the eye is rendered permanently blind.

In every type of abnormal eye condition, and especially in cataract, it is important to have the case early to secure the best results. As cataract is nearly always the result of eye strain over a period of years, it takes several months of treatment to get good results.

High degrees of presbyopia are always dangerous, for these people may develop cataract very quickly, if they are subjected to a severe nervous strain. Great worry or grief may develop a cataract in a few months.

For those who are sufficiently interested in their eyes to give some time to bringing the vision back to normal, the finest preventative for cataract is these reconstructive exercises. If they are performed even moderately, the lens will have no occasion to break down as there will be no strain on it. If glasses have been worn for a long time and their strength is excessive, a moderate amount of exercise will permit the fitting of weaker glasses.

In people past the age of muscular resiliency, this method

used together with their glasses will give clear vision long after the usual time.

In every case, the intent and ultimate result of this method is to provide the best vision possible as long as possible, freeing old age from the burden and fear of failing vision and ultimate blindness. It is always prophylactic as well as curative.

For every person who fears cataract but has not yet reached that stage, conscientious adherence to the rules of normal sight and to the practice of the simple exercises provided, offers complete relief both to the mind and to the eye.

One who has an early case of cataract may be assured that the condition may be arrested if sufficient care is taken of the eye, and the general health and habits of the individual are not inimical to satisfactory treatment. Immediate efforts should be directed toward securing perfect performance of the eye as outlined in the three rules of normal sight and the exercises for perpetuating these functions be persisted in for months. The results will more than compensate for the amount of time and energy spent in this direction.

If the cataract is complete and your surgeon feels that you have a good chance for a successful result, it may be advisable to have one eye operated upon and then observe the rules of normal sight to regain all the vision and accommodation possible in the operated eye. Should the operation be unsuccessful, I would urge anyone to spend a year trying to regain the vision in the unoperated eye before submitting to an operation on the remaining eye.

The practical results in the cases of cataract treated have been such that no one with this condition should feel himself helpless before it, but should feel encouraged that there is this modern method to be used to great benefit.

It is a popular idea that cataract is synonymous with blindness, but that is not true, and the terror that is induced by this belief should be abandoned and the condition met with intelligent, effective treatment as soon as possible.

TREATMENT FOR CATARACT

1. The extreme tension of cataract requires frequent short rest periods. Palming is the most effective means of relaxing the eyes while resting them. Place yourself in a comfortable position with something on which to rest your elbows. Cover your eyes with the palms of your hands. The hands are cupped and do not touch the eyes, the palms are on the cheekbones and the fingers of one hand crossed over the fingers of the other, without any light coming through and without pressure anywhere, no tenseness in hands or eyes. (See illustration for position of hands over eyes.) The eyes are kept softly closed. When they are completely relaxed, the background of the eye is black. The time required for this to

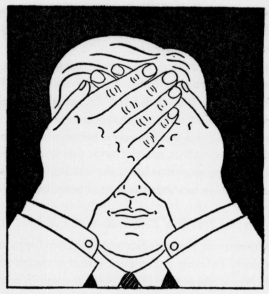

ILLUSTRATION NO. 10
Palming

take place varies from two minutes to ten minutes and, in some cases, it requires weeks of practice before a clear perception of absolute black is attained. No attempt should be made to see black. Pay no attention to the eye but occupy the mind with pleasant, quiet thoughts and the eye will take care of itself. Black appears automatically when the eye and mind are relaxed.

Palming is beneficial in all cases of eye strain as a means of resting the eyes as much as possible in as short a time as possible. A person with cataract should palm a few minutes every hour.

2. The active treatment and exercises for cataract are the same as for Middle Age Sight. Go through the exercises exactly as directed. The first seven items should be done for at least one month before any attempt is made to exercise the eyes for the near-point.

3. The Long Swing (Chapter Nine, Page 62) is the best exercise for this condition and should be done at least an hour a day. The exercises may be gone through for short periods, or one or two longer periods. The glasses must be left off or radically reduced in strength. As glasses do not help the vision much in this condition, leaving them off is no hardship.

4. Improvement in vision will continue as the exercises are performed for a period of six months to a year, or more.

5. It is best for anyone with this condition to seek the aid of a physician familiar with this method.

XVII

GLAUCOMA

Glaucoma is a condition in which the pressure of the fluids in the eyes increases above the normal to such an extent that it interferes with accommodation. In addition to this interference in accommodation, the increased pressure prevents the normal flow of blood to the retina and a gradual degeneration begins. If this is allowed to continue, the retina is destroyed and permanent blindness results.

The pressure of the fluids in the eye is kept in balance by their rate of secretion and escape through minute openings. Since any strain on the eyes increases the tension of the eye muscles, this fluid balance is interfered with. Because these fluids are not allowed to secrete and escape freely, the pressure in the eye increases and this is called glaucoma. Inflammatory and disease conditions also cause glaucoma.

The wearing of glasses for this condition is of no avail. The only relief the old method offered was surgical, and while this prevented the increases in pressure and relieved the intense pain, the degeneration of the retina continued and the operation itself caused so much damage to the eye that normal vision was impossible afterward.

The acute attacks of glaucoma almost invariably occur during the night when one is awakened with pain in the eyes, so intense that one is frequently rushed into an operation to relieve the unbearable condition.

The modern method of eye treatment is singularly successful in treating glaucoma since the entire cause of the trouble is tension.

All our automatic nerve centers have a tendency toward habit. They want to function in the same manner day after day. If you are accustomed to eating at a certain time each day, then you become hungry at that time. If you go to bed regularly, you want to go to sleep at the usual time. If you eat fast as a general thing, then eating fast becomes a habit unless consciously checked. The eyes are likewise subject to this desire to have habits.

Fortunately, there are few circumstances that produce the excessive, continuous strain that results in glaucoma. There is, nevertheless, one state where the strain is sufficient to cause this condition and that, strangely enough, is while you sleep. In order to relax completely, eyes must be allowed to move, just as you must be allowed to move in your bed or you will become tense—all muscles must move or they are held rigid. Since this is so, a normal eye moves in its socket lazily and easily and rhythmically all night.

If for any reason—such as excessive nervousness, habitual fear or tension — this unconscious movement in sleep is stopped, absolute fixation or staring ensues. If this continues, the habit of staring in one's sleep is formed and glaucoma results.

Some people, due to chronic habit of staring during their wakeful hours, have a chronic degree of glaucoma. If one uses his eyes and strains before going to bed, this same strain may be continued all night and the eyes are tired or sore or both in the morning.

On the other hand, if one does not strain but shifts normally and uses the eyes in an easy, lazy, relaxed manner, the same conditions are inclined to persist during sleep and the eyes are clear, rested, and at their best in the morning.

If the eyes are found to be strained or uncomfortable on waking, this should be sufficient warning that all is not well with them. After a six to ten hours' sleep they should feel strong and comfortable and clear. If they do not, it is positive proof that they have not been relaxed and therefore they did not rest.

A single, simple exercise, The Long Swing, (Chapter Nine,

Page 62) performed just before retiring, will correct this condition of staring in your sleep, but permanent freedom from glaucoma is secured only when normal habits of using the eyes are acquired and the eyes kept in a relaxed state all the time. Good eye habits must be used *all the time,* not just while exercising but habitually.

TREATMENT FOR GLAUCOMA

The treatment for glaucoma is the same as for cataract. Since in many cases of glaucoma the eyes stare more at night than at any other time, the Long Swing just before going to bed is most essential. This should be done from fifteen minutes to an hour, depending upon the severity of the condition. It will always give relief if taken long enough.

Placing a towel, dipped in hot water, over the eyes helps to relax them and to restore the lymphatic drainage, also to relieve the pain.

The eyes should not be used at anything requiring much concentration or for long periods at a time.

It is wise to be under the care of a physician familiar with this work who may give specific advice for this condition.

XVIII

INFLAMED EYES

Inflammation of the eyes and the margins of the eyelids is a frequent symptom of strain. This may be the result of too little sleep and exhaustion, or it may be from faulty use of the eyes such as straining to see distant objects or staring when reading.

The correction of the condition is extremely simple. The treatment outlined under the heading "Strain" will give almost immediate relief. Relaxation of the tissues in and around the eyes improves the circulation of the blood and lymph and relieves the inflammation.

Eye washes may be used to advantage when one has been in dusty, grimy, or smoky places. Boracic acid water is a safe and effective way to cleanse the eyes and may be used repeatedly as it is non-irritating. A teaspoonful to a quart of water. A normal solution of table salt (one teaspoonful to a quart of water) is also a very good, non-irritating eye wash and, since it is always available, a comfortably warm solution may be made fresh each time it is required. The warmth relaxes the eye and is soothing to the tissues.

If the eye is smarting from wind burn or the glare of light upon water or any form of irritation that can not be relieved by a simple cleansing solution, you may use murine or collyrium which may be purchased at any drug store and is very effective when used according to directions.

I would not advise the use of these as a routine matter or daily habit, as in the case of salt or boracic acid solutions, but only when necessary. There are numerous solutions put out by beauty experts which in general should be classed under the latter heading and used only when the occasion demands.

The best eye wash is made in the eye itself. Tears. This salty fluid is being made continuously and is always available when required. The lachrymal gland is under the upper lid. Frequent blinking distributes this fluid over the eye and keeps it constantly bathed. Any circumstance causing the eye to smart will be alleviated by frequent blinking. When your eyes are in difficulty from smoke, dust, or wind, nature immediately supplies more fluid to ease the condition. All that is necessary for immediate relief is to use your own remedy which you have stored in your gland. Blinking does it.

Severe inflammation of the eyes should have a diagnosis by a physician, as some eye inflammations are infectious and contagious and require local treatment.

CASE HISTORY

Inflamed Eyes
  Age 32.

History. Glasses at age of ten, and worn continuously. Increased in strength every few years. Eyes had been red with the margins of the lids red for past three years. Had used washes and drops with no permanent relief. Trouble was increasing and the eyes smarted and burned if used for a long time at one thing.

Examination showed a high degree of myopic astigmatism. Degree of vision 20/200. Unable to read without glasses unless the print was held six inches from the eyes. Retina appeared normal, also the optic nerve and blood vessels.

Treatment for myopia was given, with the glasses left off while practicing with the Snellen test card at a distance of six feet. After two weeks of treatment the glasses were changed and a much weaker lens prescribed. At the end of three weeks the eyes were clear, the margin of the lids normal and the eyes comfortable for all uses.

Note. This patient could have secured good vision without glasses if the exercises had been kept up for several months, but was interested only in getting comfort and clearing up the inflammation, so was discharged when this was accomplished.

APPENDIX

The eye is an organ composed of three layers of membrane, a tough, inelastic outer layer called the sclera, a middle layer, where the blood vessels are, called the choroid, and a third, or inmost, layer called the retina.

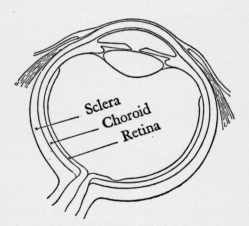

Placed in a bony depression of the skull, the shape of the cavity is large in front and smaller as it goes back into the head. The depression, immediately back of the eye, is filled with fat, giving the eye a cushion on which to turn.

Six muscles operate the eye and are attached in the front to the sclera (the outer layer of membrane) and in the back to a small bony opening at the back of the cavity or depression. Four of the muscles, called the recti muscles, pass directly back to the opening, one on each side of the eyeball, one on the top and one on the bottom. The two remaining

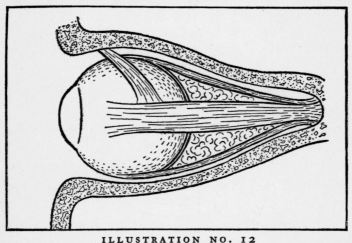

ILLUSTRATION NO. 12

The eyeball and its position in the bony cavity of the head with its muscle attachments.

muscles, called the oblique, pass partly around the eyeball, one starting from the top and the other from the bottom. They then go through a ligamentous loop or pulley before they finally go to the back of the cavity where they attach themselves to the bony opening along with the other four.

Held forward in position by the fatty pad, the eye can be operated in any direction by the four recti muscles. The purpose of the oblique muscles is to exert pressure around the middle of the eyeball, giving it power to see at varying distances by squeezing the eye and so changing the balance of pressure. When the oblique muscles are tightened, the eyeball is elongated. When the recti muscles are tightened the eyeball is shortened and thickened. This changing balance gives us our change of focus.

The sclera protects the eye against all external injury and gives it its clear white color. Four-fifths of the sclera is opaque and does not allow any light at all to penetrate. The remaining one-fifth is a translucent area, called the cornea, directly at the front in the center of the eye. It appears to be colored because of the pigment back of it, but it is in reality perfectly colorless.

The choroid, or second coat, is the blood vessel layer. It is an interwoven tissue of veins and arteries and is like a nourishing lining to the sclera, which has no blood vessels and must absorb its nourishment from the surrounding tissues. These veins and arteries in the choroid perform for the eye the same functions they perform for the other organs in the body, namely, the arteries bring to the eyes the blood so necessary for its functions and for the repair of its tissues and the veins remove the blood after it has performed this service and carry off the waste products that are left.

The third layer, the retina—in shape like a lining to the second layer—is the inner office where the real work is done. It contains all those sensitive elements which transpose light vibrations to nerve impulses, which, in turn, carry the news along the optic nerve to the visual centers in the brain.

The eye is divided front to back, into two chambers. In the front chamber is the crystalline lens with its ligament and muscle. It is, indeed, this lens that divides the eye into the two chambers, the front one being one-fifth as large as the back one. The crystalline lens is biconvex in shape and is suspended from its ligament near the front of the eye, at the junction of the cornea and the sclera.

This anterior chamber or small front room is filled with a clear water-like fluid called the aqueous humor. This fluid is being constantly created and will be replaced if lost through operation or injury. There are two very small openings or canals in this room that allow the aqueous fluid to escape. The balance between the rate of production of the aqueous humor and the rate of escape controls the amount of inner pressure you have in your eye. Pressure in the eye is necessary to maintain its shape as a perfect sphere. It is only when the eye is a perfect sphere that one can see perfectly. For many reasons it is essential that this pressure be neither too great nor too small.

There is, also, suspended in this anterior chamber, another essential structure to the intricate business of seeing—the iris. In its center is a hole, called the pupil, an empty passageway for light to pass through. It is the window through which the brain sees.

The iris performs the same function for the eye that the shutter does for the camera. It is made up of circular and radiating muscle fibers that allow it to change the size of the hole in its center so that the proper amount of light may be allowed to pass into the rear chamber to meet the needs of the eye under varying conditions.

The inner lining of the posterior chamber is, as I have said, the retina. On the back of the retina is the layer of pigment which gives the iris its color. Without this layer our eyes would have no color. In fact, it is here, on the back of the retina, that most of the pigment for the skin and hair is generated.

This delicate third coat of the eye is lightly attached to the second coat and held in place partly by a semi-fluid, semi-jelly substance called the vitreous humor. This humor fills all of this posterior room and is the other substance that helps to keep the eye a perfect sphere. Without the vitreous humor, the eye would collapse as does a rubber ball when the air is removed. Unlike the aqueous humor, if this humor is lost, it can not be replaced.

The pressure within the eye is constant, maintained by the

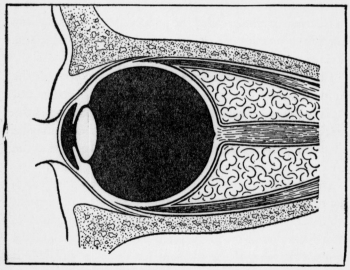

ILLUSTRATION NO. 13

The fluids of the eye are shown in black. The small body at the left is the Aqueous Humor and the large black area is Vitreous Humor. The two being separated by the Crystalline Lens.

balance between the secretion and escape of the aqueous humor. If the tension or pull of the four recti muscles is increased, the eyeball is flattened in its anterior-posterior dimensions, that is, from front to back. This is what takes place when the eye focuses for distant objects.

If, on the other hand, the tension of the oblique muscles is increased, the eye is squeezed around the middle and is elongated from front to back. This is what takes place when the eye focuses for the near point, as in reading.

When the eye is a perfect sphere and the rays of light come to a focus on the retina, a clear image is produced and one sees perfectly. When, because of tension, the rays come to a focus in front of the retina, or back of it, the image is blurred.

Light rays are refracted or bent when they pass from a media of one density to a media of another density. Before light can reach the retina, it must pass through the cornea, aqueous humor, crystalline lens, vitreous humor.

If you will look at your kodak and notice the distance adjustments on it that give you a clear image at twenty and then fifty feet, you will see how very little the eyeball needs to alter its shape in order to maintain a clear focus. This is especially so when you consider your focal lengths. The focal length in a small camera is six or seven inches, while in the eye the focal length is only about one and one-eighth inches. Some of the new small cameras, called universal focus cameras, have taken advantage of this knowledge which the study of the eye has given us and do not have to have any distance adjustment.

The varying intensity of light stimulates the retinal elements in much the same way a sensitized plate is affected in a camera. The retina of the eye is frequently compared to a photographic plate but it has some outstanding differences. The retina is composed of ten very thin layers. It would be natural to expect the seeing elements, called rods and cones, to be placed on top, composing the first layer, but this is not the case. They are, as a matter of fact, in the ninth layer and the light must pass through the first eight layers of blood vessels, nerve fibers and other thin, regular, cellular layers, before it reaches the active seeing element in the ninth layer.

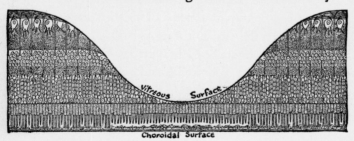

ILLUSTRATION NO. 14

The fovea centralis or spot of clear vision. The area of the fovea in the eye is the size of the head of an ordinary pin.

There is one outstanding exception to this and this is the fovea centralis, the small central spot, the size of the head of an ordinary pin, where the upper eight layers are missing and the rods and cones are exposed to the light.

There is one part of the retina on which there is no vision. On the nasal side of each eye near the middle of the back, the optic nerve passes through the three layers of the eye. The point where it enters the eyeball is a blind spot, present in every eye. It is blind because the retina does not cover this area.

As the outer side of one eye matches up with the inner side of the other eye to make one whole image when two eyes are used to see, the blind spot is never noticed, although anyone having only one eye may notice it.

The retina has two distinct types of vision. The first type is the central vision, which is the positive, clear vision, possible only in the center of the eye. This is an exceedingly small area of the retina, in fact, no larger than an ordinary pinhead. The second type is collateral vision or vision only to the extent of the general form, general motion and color. This takes up all the rest of the retina. This vision is progressively reduced, beginning at the center outward until at the periphery it is very poor indeed.

The nerve elements forming the optic nerve, after passing out of the eyeball, pass backward into the brain cavity. The nerve from the right eye does not pass directly to the right side of the brain. Soon after entering the brain cavity it splits in two and the fibers from the right side of the right eye pass to the right side of the brain and the fibers from the left side of the right eye pass to the left side of the brain. In this man-

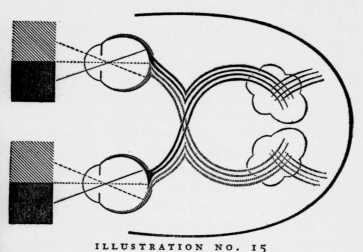

ILLUSTRATION NO. 15

The course of the nerve fibers from each eye to the brain centers. Half of the vision from each eye is carried to each lobe of the brain as illustrated.

ner each side of the brain has the fibers from half of each eye.

Millions of nerve fibers join these two centers in the brain and fuse the two images into the single image we are accustomed to seeing. When the brain is injured and this function is interfered with, double vision is produced. It is produced also when any injury to the eye muscles causes the eye to be directed improperly so that they do not co-ordinate but are directed in separate directions. This does not happen in chronic cases as the mind gradually adjusts itself to the condition and suppresses one image.

From this it is seen that the sense of vision is far from being a simple function but is made up of the accurate co-ordination of all parts of the seeing mechanism, namely, the eye, the optic nerve, and the visual centers of the brain. All these must function properly before one can see normally.